MW00843745

Just Diagnosed with

METASTATIC PANCREATIC CANCER

First Steps and More

by

Earl J. Campazzi, Jr., M.D., M.P.H., M.B.A.

with a Foreword

by

Bob Wright

Founder and Chairman, Suzanne Wright Foundation
Cofounder, Autism Speaks
Former Vice-Chairman, General Electric
Former CEO and Chairman, NBC and NBCUniversal

SERIES NOTICE,
Suzanne Wright Foundation, Publisher
610 Fifth Avenue, Suite 605
New York, NY 10020

Just Diagnosed with™

METASTATIC PANCREATIC CANCER

First Steps and More

Sandra J. Judd
Editor

Gregory J. Del Deo
Cover Designer and Illustrator

Lia N. Love
Production Editor and Title Page Designer

This book contains information that is intended to help the readers be better-informed consumers of health care. It is presented as general advice on health care and its related financial aspects, including health insurance. This book and the e-book are not intended to be a substitute for the medical advice of a licensed physician, the legal advice of an attorney, or the professional advice of a financial planner. Always consult your doctor for your individual needs about any matters relating to your health or illness.

Limit of Liability/Disclaimer of Warranty: While the publisher and author have used their best efforts in the preparation of this book, they make no representations or warranties with respect to the accuracy and completeness of the contents of this book and specifically disclaim any implied warranties or merchantability or fitness for a particular purpose. No warranty may be created or extended by sales representatives or written sales materials. The advice and strategies herein may not be suitable for your situation. You should consult with a professional where appropriate. Neither the publisher nor author shall be liable for any loss of profit or any other commercial damages, including but not limited to special, incidental, consequential, or other damages. Readers should be aware that internet websites offered as citations and/or sources for further information may have changed or disappeared between the time this was written and when it was read.

Copyright © 2017 Earl J. Campazzi, Jr., M.D., M.P.H., M.B.A.
All rights reserved. No part of this book or e-book
may be used or reproduced by any means—graphic, electronic,
or mechanical, including photocopying, recording, or taping or by any information-storage
retrieval system—without the written permission of the publisher, except in the
the case of brief quotations embodied in critical articles and reviews.

Library of Congress Control Number: 201791158
Earl J. Campazzi Jr., M.D., West Palm Beach, Florida

ISBN: 0999195603
ISBN: 9780999195604 paperback
ISBN: 978-0-9991956-1-1 e-book

Earl J. Campazzi, Jr., M.D.
Campazzi Concierge Medical Services
251 Royal Palm Way, Suite 100A
Palm Beach, FL 33480-4359

(561) 440-8879
drc@campazzi.com
www.campazzi.com

This book is dedicated to Mrs. Suzanne Wright, who died of metastatic pancreatic cancer on Friday, July 29, 2016.

Suzanne Wright is known to many for her signature achievement of cofounding Autism Speaks, the leading autism research and advocacy nonprofit organization. Those of us who knew Suzanne remember her warmth, passionate support of others, and clear sense of right and wrong. She was highly effective and unstoppable when helping others.

Acknowledgments

I am so grateful to Bob Wright, Liz Feld, and Susan Keenan of the Suzanne Wright Foundation (a.k.a. CodePurple) for supporting this book. They lent their credibility to this first-time author. CodePurple's underwriting of the printing cost will lead to wider distribution and, hopefully, greater impact. I congratulate the whole team at CodePurple for their work on behalf of the underserved pancreatic cancer patients.

Five friends and colleagues took an inordinate amount of time to guide, edit, and add content with you, the readers, in mind. Dr. Dana R. Krumholz has many years of experience as a practicing hospice and palliative-care physician. Dr. Allyson Ocean is an Associate Professor of Medicine, Hematology, and Medical Oncology at Weill Cornell Medical College, and co-founder of Let's Win PC (www.letswinpc.org). Jon S. Saxe, JD, LLM, is a very experienced pharmaceutical and biotechnology executive who has served as a director of over twenty-five companies and is a director of three public companies. Dr. Nicholas S. Aradi is a practicing psychotherapist who specializes in cognitive behavioral therapy. He sees cancer patients and their families in Palm Beach Gardens, Florida. Dr. Gregory E. Merti is my medical-school classmate and the medical director for Sentara Health Plans, a health insurer.

A special thank-you goes to Dr. Bert Vogelstein of Johns Hopkins, who took time on a Saturday to clarify the current state of genetic testing's ability to guide drug choices. He is Director of the Ludwig Center, Clayton Professor of Oncology and Pathology, and a Howard Hughes Medical Institute investigator at the Johns Hopkins Medical School and Sidney Kimmel Comprehensive Cancer Center.

Sandra J. Judd gave excellent and challenging editorial criticism. Through common-sense questions and suggestions of sections to rewrite and other aspects to explore, Sandy made remarkable contributions to shape the final version.

Editorial Services of Los Angeles provided expert and timely line editing and proofreading. Some of their work was given pro bono in support of pancreatic cancer patients. This is greatly appreciated.

Gregory J. Del Deo is a commercial artist extraordinaire. His illustrations, book jacket design, and graphics speak for themselves. As I kept changing ideas and details, Greg proved himself to be extremely professional and very patient. I recommend him highly. His email address is deldeo@gmail.com.

Incoming high-school senior and likely future doctor Lia Love is a star. She chose the font, font size, book size, and type of paper. Lia also formatted the entire book, created the title page, and took the family photo.

Last but most, the love and support of my wife, Julie, guided me through this project. Julie is not only beautiful but also an intelligent, strong, and creative woman.

Contents

Foreword

n October 2015, my wife, Suzanne, was diagnosed with stage IV pancreatic cancer. Dr. Earl Campazzi was with us from the first days of diagnosis. As we realized what Suzanne was facing, so too did we realize that all patients deserve a fierce advocate like Earl. Like other newly diagnosed patients, we were stunned by the lack of effective treatments and wondered why the cancer had gone undetected for so long. We knew pancreatic cancer was a tough one, but we had no idea we were up against *the beast*. Around the clock, I read everything published about pancreatic cancer research, and there was no good news. With a 91 percent mortality rate, why isn't this disease a federal research priority? Where is the urgency? I needed to do something. Before Suzanne died in July 2016, I promised her I would work to change the trajectory of pancreatic cancer and improve the odds for future patients.

In Suzanne's honor, I launched CodePurple, an initiative dedicated to increasing and accelerating pancreatic cancer research through awareness. We learned through our work with autism that the most effective way to drive urgency and action is through awareness. With such a tiny community of survivors, one critical role for CodePurple is to serve as a loud voice for this disease.

Without an early detection test for pancreatic cancer, 85 percent of patients are diagnosed after metastasis. Medical advances have saved millions of lives. The mammogram became a recommended screening tool for breast cancer in 1976, the PSA test was approved to detect prostate cancer in 1986, and the colonoscopy became the favored early-detection test for colon cancer in 1990. These technologies have contributed to the dramatic improvement in survival rates for these cancers. For all of this time, pancreatic cancer patients have been left behind.

This challenge demands a bold, new approach in which we measure effectiveness by lives saved, and we report results. We need to leverage private sector innovation with federal research assets to accelerate the development of an early detection test and curative treatments. High-impact research needs sizable grants with clear deliverables. Large-scale investments in medical research by Google, IBM Watson, Microsoft, and other innovators offer more promise than ever in disease detection, diagnosis, and treatment. These businesses apply their "Think Big" strategies and state-of-the-art technology to solve massive healthcare problems. This is the energy and expertise we need working on pancreatic cancer.

The National Institutes of Health (NIH) and the National Cancer Institute (NCI) conduct essential basic research for breakthroughs in all diseases. However, with no progress in nearly fifty years, pancreatic cancer clearly requires a different approach focused on translational science and the best technology available. In the 1990s, the NIH partnered with the Defense Advanced Research Project Agency (DARPA), NASA, and the CIA to use their advanced imaging technology for dramatic improvement in breast cancer screening. We must treat pancreatic cancer with urgency, effective leadership, and the level of priority it demands to save lives.

The federal government has committed to innovation, and the landscape has been primed for a bold new approach to pancreatic cancer research. Bipartisan congressional support for innovation makes a pilot program for pancreatic cancer both viable and promising.

If you are reading this book, pancreatic cancer has affected you or someone you love. The best way to make progress is to make your voice heard. Please join us in our fight against pancreatic cancer, and visit our website: Codepurplenow.org.

Bob Wright
Spring 2017

Preface

With this book, it is my hope to give you a realistic overview of your difficult challenge with metastatic pancreatic carcinoma. The fifteen action steps are designed to be practical and easily read in one sitting. This book is purposely short, as you are probably overwhelmed. The appendices A through D provide additional information, and I have also included references.

My intention is not to give specific advice or answer all questions because each patient is different. Rather, I want to offer some guidance to help you navigate the medical system. I include the following:

1. Questions to ask

2. Options to consider

3. Yellow flags (proceed with caution)

4. Red flags (suggest making a change)

Recommendations will vary depending on your specific situation at any given time. Therefore, this book does not include a list of specific physicians, medical centers, or vendors.

I have always felt the need to practice medicine in the *real world*, considering disabilities, differing languages, and varying economic resources among patients. Greater resources will certainly allow patients to procure more assistance, testing, and review by additional experts. However, even if you have all the money in the world, there is no cure for metastatic pancreatic cancer that you can buy.

To the extent possible, I seek to democratize cancer treatment by suggesting ways to get comprehensive care despite financial constraints. A lack of resources usually necessitates more work of various types. For instance, finding and applying for charitable funds and clinical trials is quite time-consuming.

The dollar-sign notations below give general patient financial categories. Later, costs of supplementary treatments, additional testing and imaging, and second opinions are matched to these categories.

$ Paying the insurance deductible and copayment costs can cause economic hardship. The partial, or likely total, reduction in income caused by the patient's illness will add to that economic stress. At best, several hundred dollars would be available to pay out-of-pocket for care or testing not covered by insurance.

$$ In addition to paying the necessary costs associated with pancreatic cancer, there would be $1,000 to $10,000 available to spend wisely and carefully on supplementary treatments, additional testing and imaging, and second opinions.

$$$ Out-of-pocket expenditures for pancreatic cancer treatments are possible but cannot be unlimited. The amount available would be $10,000 to $100,000.

$$$$ There is virtually no limit on the out-of-pocket expenditures if there is some potential for benefit. There is also the possibility of contributing to pancreatic cancer research or a charitable organization.

This book is designed to be read very soon after you are diagnosed with metastatic pancreatic cancer. If you have nonmetastatic (localized) cancer, or if you have already started treatment, recommendations about teams, organization, and supplemental tests and treatments still apply to you.

I am listing pertinent search terms for internet searches. Presumably, the relevance of these terms will remain almost constant even as the search results change over time because of scientific advances. The list of search terms should extend the usefulness of this book. (See Appendix B.)

The introduction includes a discussion of insurance considerations. Understanding how insurance works may be essential toward optimizing care. Also, in Appendix D, you will find a glossary of some medical terms used in this book.

Some people learn best by reading while others prefer audiovisual learning. Consequently, I give you web addresses of videos about pancreatic cancer with suggested video time ranges. Seeing diagrams and pictures will speed your learning. The audio portions will help with simple but important concepts such as the pronunciation of medical terms. The goal is for you to quickly understand your problem and formulate your plan. For your convenience, video links are listed in Appendix B and are also posted on my website, Campazzi.com. I will keep the website list updated as new videos become available.

Introduction

Metastatic pancreatic cancer is a terrible diagnosis. I do not want to give you false hope. *Yet there is hope.* Your unique path is ahead. You can benefit from those before you who volunteered for and participated in cancer research. *If you find and use all the medical and supportive care that is currently available for people with pancreatic cancer, it is likely your outcome will be better than predicted by statistics.* Significantly better, I hope.

While there is no magical cure for metastatic pancreatic cancer that is being kept a secret, I am a big believer in seeking the best possible care. The natural tendency is to focus on the gap between what is known and what is needed. This gap can only be bridged slowly and with a worldwide effort.

The gap you need to focus on is the one between your current medical care and the best that is presently available. Sadly, this difference can be quite sizable. Patients fail to seek the best care for many reasons. Among them are a bond with their doctor(s), the convenience of getting care locally, a lack of awareness of options, a lack of resources, hesitancy to travel, and fear of the unknown. There are much bigger differences than there should be between the medical care provided at the best specialty-care centers and that offered in most communities.[1] (*If you are going to read only one reference from this book, this is the one you should choose.*)

There are two overarching themes in this book. The first is that you cannot fight pancreatic cancer alone. Both practically and psychologically, this disease is a tremendous challenge, and you will need to create a team of people to help you. Ideally, your team should include family, friends, and professionals with a variety of expertise. The second theme is that you must fight pancreatic cancer with as much information as possible.

The best plan is to have a multidisciplinary team working for you. No single expert knows everything. Most specialists are focused on their own specific area(s). By putting the best minds together, amazing things can happen.

A multidisciplinary approach is used more commonly at cancer treatment centers than by community oncologists. Such an approach includes the use of truly awe-inspiring genetic testing. Many genetic tests are readily available at academic centers and commercial laboratories. New and advanced testing is being studied in clinical trials.

A practical consideration is health-insurance coverage, which varies widely among patients with pancreatic cancer. Your insurance will not necessarily cover all the care you want and need. Actually, health insurers do not promise to take the best possible care of you, but rather they commit to fulfilling their obligations under their legal contract with you. You and, perhaps, your employer pay the health insurer a certain amount, and in exchange, the insurer provides very specific benefits as detailed in their Summary of Benefits and Coverage (SB&C). This document has a variety of other similar names such as "Benefit Language" and "Evidence of Coverage."

---

1. Sharon Begley, "Why a Top Cancer Center Could Save Your Life," *Newsweek*, October 16, 2009, http://www.newsweek.com/why-top-cancer-center-could-save-your-life-81425, accessed November 1, 2016.

When originally introduced, health insurance was a way to pay for whatever medical care your doctor ordered. Those lucky enough to be healthy provided their unused funds to care for the sick. This was called *risk pooling*. While it is a term still used, the meaning of risk pooling has evolved away from insurers being passive payers.

Today, health insurers play a direct role in cancer care through selective payment. *Preauthorization* (a.k.a. *precertification*) has become a dominant concept. Although your doctor still decides what is best for you, your health insurer must preauthorize the payment for the expensive parts of your treatment.

Preauthorization not only "refers to what diagnostic and therapeutic care are pre-approved for coverage by the plan but also where and by whom the care is provided. For example, Health Maintenance Organization (HMO) patients may wish to receive care from a national center of excellence for a particular cancer only to be told that they must get all their care directly from those providers who participate in their HMO network."[2]

Health insurers contract with health providers, including doctors, laboratories, infusion centers, and hospitals. Those under contract with the health insurer are termed *in-network*. HMOs usually pay only for care given in-network. For cancer care, some HMOs provide for an out-of-network *expert* opinion, so *it is important to read your SB&C*. Pay particularly close attention to the exclusions and limitations section.

Another type of coverage is Preferred Provider Organization (PPO). It will pay for out-of-network care. However, the amount you are covered for ranges from somewhat to dramatically less than you would receive for in-network care. When the coverage is less, you have greater *direct costs*

---

2. Dr. Gregory Merti, e-mail communication to author, July 5, 2017.

(out of pocket) in the form of higher copayments and higher deductibles. Eventually, you can run into much greater direct cost after reaching *payer limit*. For many policies, there is a total amount the insurer will pay, and then you effectively have no more health insurance, at least from that company.

The standard-of-care treatment for pancreatic cancer is partly defined by what insurance companies authorize. This is usually chemotherapy, which extends life, on average, by only several months. Chemotherapy causes significant, even debilitating, side effects. Ideally, chemotherapy will not only extend your life but also provide a bridge to more effective treatment as it becomes available.

I recommend *standard-of-care plus*, which is a term and concept that I learned from Dr. Allyson Ocean. The *plus* is promising new treatments that are often not paid for by insurers. This book offers an awareness of treatment options that are beyond the standard of care, along with tools you can use to avoid overhyped and dangerous treatments.

You may eventually want to participate in clinical trials approved by the Food and Drug Administration (FDA). The good news is some insurers are now covering them—even HMOs as long the trial is being conducted in-network. Other clinical trials are financially supported by research grants or by pharmaceutical companies. Out-of-pocket costs such as travel, lodging, and meals are usually reimbursed for the patient participating in the clinical trial and one caregiver.

Depending on your insurance, you may be able to seek coverage (insurance payment) for non-standard-of-care testing and treatment. The cardinal rule in applying for these funds is to know the rules. The Patient Advocate Foundation can be a resource.[3]

---

3. Patient Advocate Foundation, Last Modified 2012, http://www.patientadvocate.org/index.php?p=757, accessed July 5, 2017.

It has been my experience that requests to receive care from out-of-network providers for medical services that are offered in-network are almost always denied. This is the case even though you perceive (even with supporting data) that these services are delivered with higher quality and have better outcomes out-of-network. Appeals for *medically needed services* (the definition of this term can be the subject of debate with your health insurer) not offered in-network are more often (but far from always) granted.

Health insurers try to make the preauthorization process clear on their websites. Further details are in the SB&C, but this document can be difficult to fully understand. It is well worth the call to the Plan Member's Services Center to get further information. Sometimes a representative will give you some valuable insight into their guidelines or decision-making process for authorizing nonstandard testing and treatment.

Preauthorizations may require an initial request from your doctor. The appeal of an initial denial can be the responsibility of either the doctor or the patient depending on the details of your insurance. Subsequent appeals are frequently the responsibility of the patient. These are often but not always denied. If you are going to be denied, you want to make sure it is because you do not qualify for the benefit rather than for a technicality of not following procedures. For example, you could have received a service that would have been covered, but you did not get the *required preauthorization.*[4]

There are also unique situations regarding employer-provided health insurance. Some companies are self-insured, so a health-insurance company functions only as the administrator of the plan. Appeals for coverage denial may be very company-specific in this case. Also, some patients are members of unions that can act as patient advocates regarding insurance coverage.

---

4. Dr. Gregory Merti, e-mail communication to author, July 5, 2017.

Even decisions regarding Medicare coverage are not perfectly straightforward. You have an option of electing for Part D of Medicare. Some chemotherapy is given intravenously and is covered by a member's medical rather than pharmacy benefit—which often has differing copays or coinsurances. Other types of chemotherapy come in pill form and are given by mouth, and these are covered by the pharmacy benefit. The decision to opt for Part D takes some thought.[5] Also, there is an additional benefit, called the Medicare Savings Program, for low-income Medicare recipients who do not necessarily qualify for Medicaid.[6]

While more testing can be done on a self-paid basis, these tests will not necessarily lead to an improved outcome. Nonetheless, such testing will provide more data about your tumor with the hope it will be advantageous. Financing additional testing or cutting-edge treatment is, unfortunately, an option for only some.

However, there are sometimes ways to afford new or experimental treatments. It can take a lot of legwork and research to find and use these resources. Options include using the life benefit of your life insurance, using benefits from your long-term care insurance, or meeting the qualifications for early withdrawal from your 401(k) or IRA. A reverse mortgage can perhaps be a consideration, but the pros and cons of it are beyond the scope of this book.

For any of the options I have listed above, you should speak to a reputable financial professional who is independent of any transaction.

---

5. American Cancer Society, Last Modified 2017, https://www.cancer.org/treatment/finding-and-paying-for-treatment/understanding-health-insurance/health-insurance-options/medicare/medicare-part-d/things-people-with-cancer-need-to-think-about.html, accessed July 5, 2017.

6. American Cancer Society, Last Modified 2017, https://www.cancer.org/treatment/finding-and-paying-for-treatment/understanding-health-insurance/health-insurance-options/medicare/medicare-part-d/getting-help-to-pay-for-medicare.html, accessed July 5, 2017.

Ideally, he or she should be compensated only for his or her professional services. Always be wary when a financial adviser recommends a transaction from which they receive a commission.

There are charitable funds designated for patient care. Even specialists at a medical center may not be aware of small donations that have been designated for clinical care. It is up to you to find the appropriate office or person to ask. Many of these funds are available for medical care only at a specific medical center.

For the many with modest financial means, I suggest asking family and friends to provide financial assistance for treatment not covered by insurance. You might also want to try crowdfunding. This works particularly well through an internet registry, especially if you are a member of a close-knit group such as a religious community, police, or firefighters. You will be surprised how many will help you get the best medical care possible!

Staying on the money theme for a moment, think of your health like your money. You can have professionals, friends, and family advising you. Yet ultimately you have primary responsibility for your own medical care, just as you do for your life savings.

Except in an emergency, your doctors should present you with all relevant information and options. You should be empowered to direct your own care or to delegate that choice to a surrogate to decide for you. He or she is generally instructed to make choices based on your preferences and beliefs.

Pancreatic cancer is disempowering and overwhelming. To make the needed weighty decisions, bear in mind the following:

1. There is a tremendous benefit to having all your information about pancreatic cancer organized.

2. You should double-check virtually everything you are told due to the seriousness of the disease.

3. Throughout the course of your disease, you and your team should passionately gather information, as the body of relevant science is rapidly growing and evolving.

4. Your physician should welcome thoughtful questions that stem from your research.

Basics About Your Pancreas and Pancreatic Cancer

Your pancreas is a six-inch organ that looks like an upside-down hot chili pepper. Here it is shown with and without a tumor.

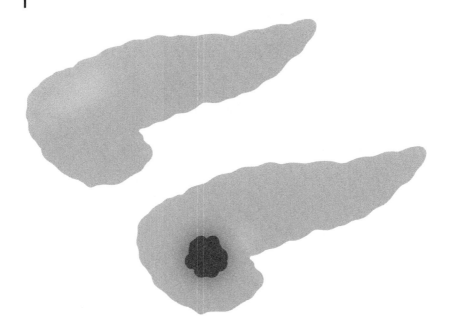

Your pancreas helps you digest food and regulates your glucose (sugar) level. It lies at a diagonal behind the stomach and below your breastbone (sternum). The head of the pancreas is slightly past the midline on your right side, where its tail slopes upward to the left, behind your stomach, and is protected by your lower left ribs.

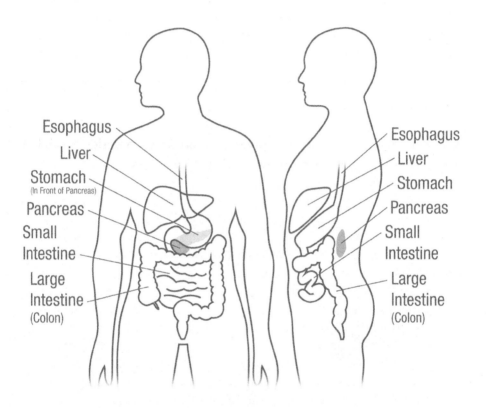

Esophagus
Liver
Stomach
(In Front of Pancreas)
Pancreas
Small
Intestine
Large
Intestine
(Colon)

Esophagus
Liver
Stomach
Pancreas
Small
Intestine
Large
Intestine
(Colon)

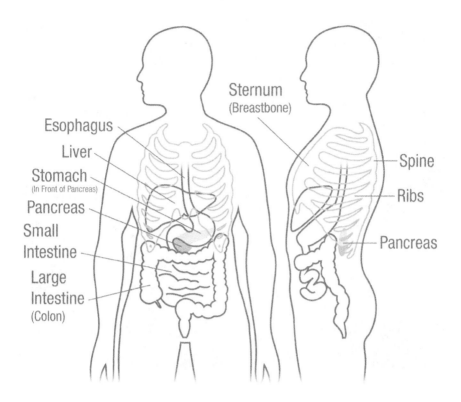

A significant challenge with the pancreas is that it is nearly in the center of the body. For diagnosis and treatment of pancreatic cancer, the pancreas is in a simply terrible position. Because the pancreas is so deep inside the body (front to back), it is hard to for a doctor to feel it when examining a patient.

Unfortunately, neither the patient nor his or her doctor is usually aware of a growing mass in the pancreas until it is quite large. Surgery and radiation therapy for pancreatic cancer are also technically difficult because of its location and the large arteries (high-pressure blood vessels) near it.

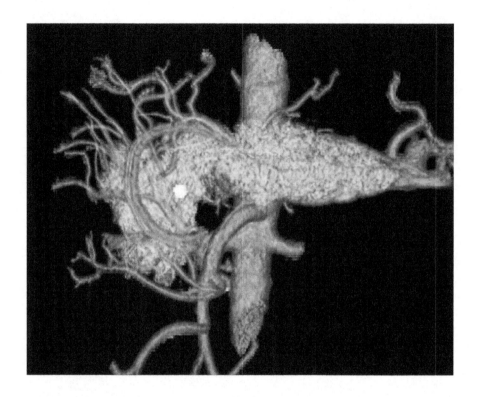

Let's take a step back and look at the whole body because a basic understanding will help you as you make decisions about treatment. *The body is so complex that it is a miracle it works at all.* Logically, something so complex is not simple to treat. Keep your guard up when you hear of simple cancer cures. Virtually every treatment has unintended consequences, or symptoms called side effects.

Visualize the body as if you are looking at a Google map that has four levels of magnification. These levels of focus vary markedly. Imagine the difference between a view of the whole earth, a map of your state, a map of your neighborhood, and a view that will allow you to read license plates and identify people. With that in mind, here are our four levels of magnification as applied to the body:

- **Whole person:** The whole care team needs to keep in mind that they are *treating a person with pancreatic cancer, not simply* *pancreatic cancer!* Any treatment of cancer must also concern itself with the health and well-being of the person as a whole. This is a reminder to also look through the broadest lens first.

- **The organs:** The body has various parts called organs that can be seen only with imaging (x-ray, ultrasound, CT, or MRI) or in surgery. They are like departments of the body, as each does just a few jobs. A few of these organs are absolutely necessary to keep living. You can live without your pancreas, which is causing you so much trouble, but not without your liver. The liver, where pancreatic cancer often spreads, is essential to life because it detoxifies the body.

   Notably, the liver is very resilient. The liver can function with metastases from pancreatic cancer, even if they are numerous and large. However, there can come the point when pancreatic cancer causes the liver to fail. Unfortunately, a liver transplant is not an option to treat pancreatic cancer because it would not cure your pancreatic cancer. A new liver would soon have metastases and would fail. Liver failure is a frequent cause of death from pancreatic cancer.

- **The cells:** Cells are the smallest structures of your body. They can be seen only with a microscope. There are approximately *one trillion cells in the human body*—the number of drops of water in one thousand swimming pools. The body is clearly a very complex system.

- **DNA:** DNA is the *secret code* that directs our cells. It contains all the biological information that makes us all who we are. There are three billion DNA base pairs (like the zero or one bits of information in digital technology) in each and every cell. Every cell contains as many DNA codes as there are drops of water in three swimming pools. So, when a DNA mutation causes cancer in millions of cells, controlling the disease is an enormous challenge.

Science fiction is another way to explain pancreatic cancer. Think of a pancreatic cell as a spaceship in the galaxy of the body. Like a large spacecraft of the future, these cells are as busy as a city inside. Mostly, cells are *reading* their DNA codes to make proteins of three types:

- **Enzymes:** They function like mindless robots. After it is released by a pancreatic cell, each enzyme does only one thing but does it over and over again. For instance, some enzymes cut the protein we eat into small pieces, and others carve up the fat.

- **Hormones:** These proteins are "exported" into your blood by some of your pancreatic cells. Hormones are messengers to other cells. For instance, the hormone insulin is made by the pancreas and will be discussed later.

- **Cell-surface markers:** These are proteins that are made to stay on the surface of cells, including pancreatic cells. There are two general types of cell markers.
    a. *Identification markers:* Like an ID badge, these proteins tell the immune cells not to attack pancreatic cells because they are part of the body.
    b. *Hormone receptors:* Pancreatic cancer cells also receive messages. These are like docking stations on a spacecraft.

Cancer cells are spaceships that are out of control. In addition to multiplying, pancreatic cancer cells also produce abnormal cell-surface markers. These protein markers can be used to define different types of pancreatic cancer. For instance, some types grow and spread faster than others. The differences in these abnormal cell surface proteins are very important, as some abnormal proteins can be susceptible to different cancer-fighting drugs. Therefore, your doctors should learn as much about your particular cancer cells as they can. As time goes on, medicine is evolving toward targeted therapy that will be able to specifically target *your treatment* to *your cancer*. This is called *personalized medicine* and could ultimately mean the difference between success and failure.

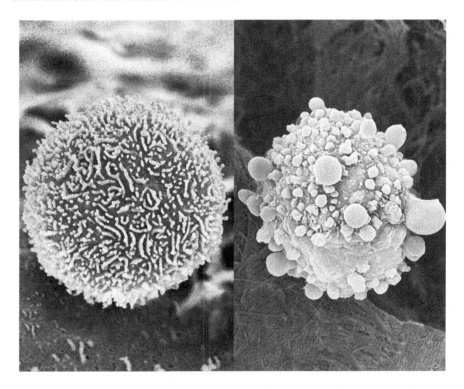

These extremely magnified images of pancreatic cancer cells make a few points. Clearly, they are not identical, thus the need for a pathologist to accurately categorize them. The cell on the left could be overproducing an ID badge-like protein that inhibits the immune system. The cell on the right appears to be growing wildly. Therefore, it could be producing a cell-surface protein (cell marker) unique to it. If so, this would be an opportunity for personalized immune therapy ($$$).

As previously mentioned, the pancreas releases the proteins it produces via two routes. Hormones are secreted directly into your blood. Enzymes reach your intestines by flowing through your pancreatic duct, which is a tube in the middle of your pancreas.

Curiously, most pancreatic cancers arise from the simple cells (called ductal cells) that form the pancreatic duct. Cancer of these cells is called adenocarcinoma, which is by far the most common type of pancreatic cancer.

Adenocarcinoma of the duct cells is that it can block the flow of digestive enzymes. Digestive enzymes can be dangerous if they build up inside the pancreas because they are little automatic scissors *designed* to robotically cut food into microparticles for digestion. When digestive enzymes build up, these mindless little scissors begin attacking the pancreas and any other tissue they can access.

To treat this, a stent (a tiny metal tube that opens and stays open like a spring) is sometimes used to keep your bile duct open. Your pancreatic duct is too small to be stented (forcibly opened) in most cases. Stenting the bile duct, which is bigger and immediately downstream, usually helps avoid enzyme buildup and its associated problems.

Late-stage ductal adenocarcinoma can also adversely affect the hormone-producing cells of the pancreas. Insulin is one of the hormones produced by the pancreas. You have most probably heard of it. The islet cells (beta cell subtype, to be exact) of the pancreas produce it. Insulin attaches to receptors on almost all cells of the body. It leads to sugar (glucose) being *carried* through the cell wall to the interior of the cell where it can be used. Think of this process like having a doorman at a hotel carrying suitcases inside.

Diabetes is a disease that can be caused by all types of pancreatic cancer. With diabetes, your insulin level is low, and blood sugar is high. Sounds good? Perhaps a little extra energy when you need it? Diabetes is just the opposite. Like luggage piling up in front of a hotel, the blood sugar we measure is outside the cell. With diabetes, the cells throughout your body begin to starve and do not function correctly. There is not enough insulin to carry sugar to where it is needed—that is, inside cells. Low-sugar diets can prevent and help treat diabetes.

I am only briefly mentioning a type of pancreatic cancer that starts in the islet cell. Acinar cell carcinoma is usually a localized (nonmetastatic) tumor and accounts for only 1 to 2 percent of all pancreatic cancers. In general, this type of cancer has a better prognosis and is treated differently from the much more common pancreatic adenocarcinoma. Surgery is often the recommended treatment. This book's general principles of forming a team, being organized and getting second opinions for multiple aspects of your care apply.

Pancreatic cancer that has not spread beyond the pancreas (nonmetastatic) is also only briefly mentioned in this book. For pancreatic cancer in this stage, surgery is sometimes technically possible. Overall, only 15 percent to 20 percent of individuals with pancreatic cancer are candidates for surgery.[7] About 25 percent of those who have surgery are cured.

Sometimes immediate surgery is recommended. Other times, chemotherapy is used to shrink the tumor to make surgery possible. For surgery to be an option, you will need to be in reasonably good health, and the tumor cannot be entwined with the major nerves or blood vessels that are very close to the pancreas.

Much further discussion of nonmetastatic cancer is planned for a future book. Again, several general concepts about how to approach pancreatic cancer detailed in this book are common to all types of pancreatic cancer.

7. "Pancreatic Cancer and Whipple Procedure", *Pancreatica*, Last Modified 2017, http://pancreatica.org/pancreatic cancer/pancreatic cancer-surgical-treatment/, accessed May 27, 2017.

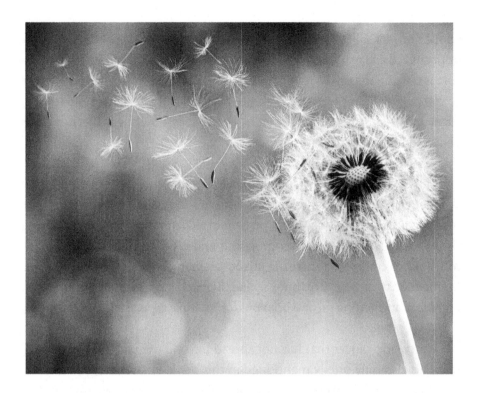

Pancreatic cancer cells can spread to other places in the body by entering the bloodstream. Almost like a seed, these cells can take root in the liver (most commonly), lung, bone, brain, or other locations. A common hope is that if the cancer that has spread, it has spread to only one part of the body but nowhere else. Unfortunately, like a dandelion in the wind, if your pancreatic cancer has metastasized at all, it has probably spread throughout your body in microscopic form. At this point, you need a type of whole-body (systemic) treatment.

Cancer is a disease that causes cells to start dividing and grow out of control. Human cells grow by splitting in two and then increasing in size. The most rapid period of human growth is before birth. Cancers grow by *turning back on* the growth genes that were used in childhood. Cancer cells divide, grow, and divide again at a furious pace.

The immune system struggles to be effective against pancreatic cancer. This is probably because pancreatic cancer creates a fibrous stroma (like a thick spider's web) microenvironment in which the cancer cells grow. The cancer cells are shielded from your immune system as if they were in a fort. See the photo on the back cover, which depicts a large amount of fibrosis.

The web encompassing your pancreatic cancer cells allows for little blood flow to the cancer cells, but "unlike any other cancer, pancreatic tumors are able to survive with a very limited blood supply."[8] Minimal blood supply helps pancreatic cancer cells resist treatment because the blood circulates chemotherapy and other medications.

8. Rachel Tompa, "Immunotherapy for Pancreatic Cancer Boosts Survival More Than 75 Percent in Mice, Study Finds," *Hutch News*, 2015, https://www.fredhutch.org/en/news/center-news/2015/10/ Immunotherapy-boosts-pancreatic cancer-survival-study-finds.html, accessed May 7, 2017, reprinted with permission.

Action Step One: Pause

There are different ways you could have learned that you have pancreatic cancer. The best scenario is having had no symptoms before an incidental finding. For example, it is possible for doctors to discover a tumor in the pancreas during a scan for gallbladder disease. When pancreatic cancer is found this way, there is good chance that it has not spread.

Unfortunately, the most common scenario is like the beginning of a roller-coaster ride. At first, you have mild symptoms such as an upset stomach. It seems like nothing, but it persists. Then you begin to worry, just as you do when starting up the first roller-coaster hill. You go to your primary care doctor. He or she orders some routine tests. The results are a little concerning, like getting higher and higher off the ground. Fear of the unknown increases as the preliminary findings necessitate a CT scan. Finding a pancreatic mass on a CT scan is the terror of starting down the first hill on a roller coaster. Everything seems out of control.

Unlike on a roller coaster, you can temporarily put on the emergency brake. You can take control of the care process and, hopefully, your cancer. Pancreatic cancer is a shocking diagnosis. You need time to digest, gather information, undergo additional testing, get second opinions, and choose your initial treatment—but not too much time.

One of the first questions that arises is the length of time to spend gathering information and seeking second opinions before beginning treatment. You should ask the physician who made your diagnosis how urgently you need treatment. If your physician initially responds with "as soon as possible," you should ask whether this is an emergency that needs treatment today or this week, or whether two weeks would be a safe and reasonable time to gather information before making a treatment decision.

The literature states that it takes approximately one decade for pancreatic cancer to begin from the one-cell stage. Of course, by the time it is clinically apparent, it is growing much faster than it was at the start. As a general guide, two weeks is often a reasonable amount of time before initiating treatment. I defer specific direction about this matter to your oncologist.

Action Step Two: Form A Care Team

After a diagnosis of metastatic pancreatic cancer, you face a complicated and physically demanding regimen of treatment. There are many decisions that will need to be made, and you will not be feeling your best. You need to build a care team of medical professionals, family, friends, and, perhaps, paid assistants to help you as you move through this process. Your care team has three missions:

1. To get you the best medical care possible

2. To keep you comfortable
   a. Minimizing symptoms, including pain, from pancreatic cancer
   b. Minimizing side effects from treatment

3. To keep you mentally healthy
   a. Watching for depression and anxiety—and treating early, if needed
   b. Giving social support
   c. Making sure your religious and spiritual needs are met

You should start by choosing a patient advocate who will be a part of your emotional support team, who will help you form the rest of your care team, and who will help you form a plan for staying organized. Your patient advocate should be the person who can help you the most. Often it will be your spouse or adult child. Alternatively, there are paid professionals who offer this service.

Your patient advocate will need to make time available and have the willingness to be heavily involved. There are other useful qualities to look for in him or her, including a calm disposition, familiarity with your likes, dislikes, family situation, and finances, and so on. Your advocate will need to have the willingness and the ability to learn details about medical treatments, alternative treatments, and insurance issues. Your choice of an advocate needs to be made reasonably quickly, so trust your instincts, and don't get bogged down here.

You do not have to announce your choice. There is no need to ruffle feathers, as there is probably already enough emotional strain on your family. Instead, you should simply encourage one person to be with you at most appointments. This is the person to chiefly rely on for counsel as treatment choices arise.

No two teams will be identical, but effective teams have certain similarities. Your team should be built quickly, as pancreatic cancer becomes overwhelming fast. The day-to-day roles and responsibilities of your care team fall into three broad categories:

1. Medical care

2. Emotional support

3. Information management

Winning teams have players with different skill sets. The number of paid professionals you will have versus how many family members and friends you must recruit will vary with the available resources. Bear in mind: *money makes you wealthy, but friends make you rich.*

The list for the medical team is long. You should start with an oncologist, a consulting oncologist(s) (second opinion(s)), and a consulting pathologist. You do not have to make appointments with everyone else on day one, but you will be surprised by how many of these physicians, nurses, and scientists you will need over time.

Medical Care Team

a. ***Oncologist***: An oncologist is a physician who has completed medical school and an additional three years of advanced training in internal medicine with further training in oncology, a subspecialty of internal medicine that focuses on treating patients with cancer. Your oncologist should not only direct your pancreatic cancer treatment but also oversee all medical care you receive.

b. ***Consulting oncologist***: You should seek one or preferably two unrelated second opinions from academic oncologists (professors of medicine at schools of medicine). They will confirm the type and subtype of pancreatic cancer that you have and suggest treatment options. There is surprising and concerning variation in quality and approach to cancer care across care providers and medical centers.

c. ***Consulting pathologist***: You would have a disaster if the foundation to your home were not laid properly. Pathology is the foundation of cancer care. A pathologist is a doctor who examines the tumor cells from your biopsy under a microscope. Through magnification and the use of different stains, he or she can tell whether your cells are cancerous or normal.

If they are cancerous, the pathologist can tell how aggressive (how quickly they are likely to grow and spread) your cancer cells are. You will probably never meet your initial pathologist, the hospital where you have your biopsy choses him or her.

Since it is essential that you have the precisely correct pancreatic cancer diagnosis, including type and subtype, from the beginning, *I suggest that you send your pathology slides (or a CD with digital images of them) to a consulting pathologist at an academic center that specializes in pancreatic cancer* ($).You should search the internet for the term *pathology second opinion*.

d. **Consulting radiologist**: A radiologist's primary responsibility is to determine if your cancer has spread. He or she reads your x-rays and CT scans and writes a report that details the size, shape, and number of your tumor(s). Depending on the imaging technique used, the radiologist can also see if your tumor is near any major blood vessels or blocking the bile or pancreatic ducts. This is another physician you probably will not meet, and your hospital chose for you.

There are radiologists who specialize in the GI (gastrointestinal) system and are very experienced with pancreatic cancer. It is easy to have your images (x-rays, ultrasounds, CT scans, or MRIs) sent to them in digital format on a CD ($$). You should conduct a web search for the term *pancreatic cancer radiology second opinion*.

e. **Geneticist**: A geneticist advises you about the rapidly progressing field of genetic testing and genetics-based treatment. He or she can also evaluate whether your relatives are at a significantly increased risk of getting pancreatic cancer, considering your diagnosis. If possible, every pancreatic cancer patient should see a geneticist ($$) before making his or her initial treatment decision. Health insurance policies often cover brief but, notably, not comprehensive genetic consults.

f. ***Primary care physician***: Your primary care physician works with your oncologist to take care of some of the side effects of pancreatic cancer and its treatments, including infections and associated dehydration. Infections are more likely when you are undergoing chemotherapy because chemotherapy weakens the immune system. If left untreated, infection in a cancer patient will quickly lead to the need for emergency care. Your primary care physician will be responsible for staying ahead of medical issues that are secondary to the cancer treatment and for preventing these issues from becoming life threatening.

Your primary care physician also will have to care for diabetes if it arises. As previously mentioned, it is common for patients with pancreatic cancer to develop diabetes because the pancreas produces insulin. Diabetes always requires medical evaluation and care from your primary care physician often with the assistance of a specialist (endocrinologist).

Medical problems unrelated to diabetes continue to need to be addressed by your primary care physician. You might have high blood pressure or thyroid disease. Since the average age of pancreatic cancer diagnosis is seventy,[9] many people with pancreatic cancer also have other health problems, which their doctor must continue to treat.

Some primary care physicians, such as those practicing on a direct-payment or concierge model, can take a larger role in your pancreatic cancer treatment ($$$). They can research and recommend specialists for second opinions. They can also evaluate alternative and supplemental treatments. Some primary care physicians become *medical care managers*, facilitating the coordination of all your specialists and specialized testing results. Primary

9. National Cancer Institute, "SEER Stat Fact Sheet: Pancreas Cancer," http://seer.cancer.gov/statfacts/html/pancreas.html, accessed November 1, 2016.

care physicians in this role can help with insurance issues. You will want to talk to your primary care physician soon after your diagnosis to determine how large a role he or she will want to play in your treatment.

g. **Palliative care physician**: Specialists in palliative medicine have a different perspective. They make suggestions to minimize pain, nausea, vomiting, night sweats and other symptoms while increasing appetite. Dr. Allyson Ocean of Weill Cornell Medicine and cofounder of Let's Win PC (letswinpc.org) suggests including palliative medicine at the very beginning of your cancer care. Her recommendation is based on her experience, which is supported by a published study.[10]

She finds that patients have better outcomes if full attention is paid to minimizing their symptoms and side effects from the beginning. Receiving palliative medicine is perfectly compatible with aggressively treating pancreatic cancer. Your palliative-care specialists will work with your treating oncologist and other physicians ($—most health-insurance policies cover palliative medicine).

h. **Home nursing ($$$)**: Nurses are very valuable for those who can afford them. Compared to twenty years ago, "people who were previously cared for in the hospital are now cared for at home."[11]

Without any regard for the patient's dignity, the symptoms of pancreatic cancer and its treatment include fatigue, mouth ulcers, nausea, vomiting, diarrhea, fecal incontinence, bloating, back and

---

10. Lynn Howie and Jeffrey Peppercorn, "Early Palliative Care in Cancer Treatment: Rationale, Evidence and Clinical Implications," *Therapeutic Advances in Medical Oncology* (November 5, 2013); 5(6): 318–23, https://www.ncbi.nlm.nih.gov/pmc/articles/PMC3799294/, accessed May 30, 2017.

11. Eileen O'Reilly and Joanne Frankel Kelvin, *100 Questions and Answers about Pancreatic Cancer*, 2nd ed. (Sudbury, MA: Jones and Bartlett Publishers, 2010), 149.

abdominal pain, dark and smelly urine, and bed-soaking sweats. While a nurse's training goes far beyond dealing with these problems, there is nothing like a sympathetic and capable nurse when you are so ill. Most prefer a nurse to a family member for hands-on assistance with bodily fluid issues.

i. ***Psychiatrists and psychologists***: It is important for cancer patients to be open to professional mental health care. Living with a diagnosis of cancer is a traumatic experience, and it is common for patients to suffer from feelings of anxiety or depression. A mental-health professional can help you deal with these feelings (and ranges from $ to $$$ depending on insurance coverage and frequency of appointments).

Though you may also have friends and family with whom you can talk, mental-health professionals offer two essential advantages over friends and family. First, they are trained in how to listen, question, and make suggestions. Second, they are compensated, so there is no sense of imposing on them. Unfortunately, pancreatic cancer creates the need for mental health care in far more patients than those who access it. Consider seeking mental health care.

j. ***Interventional radiologist***: Much like a surgeon, interventional radiologists perform procedures on the deep tissues of your body. For instance, they do minimally invasive liver biopsies, either through the skin or the jugular vein (a procedure that sounds horrible but has only rare complications). They also do the Y-90 procedure, which is discussed in "Action Step Seven." (The money code is hard to assign, as this consult, and the resulting procedures, may not be considered standard of care. $—if covered by Medicare. $$—if covered by private insurance, given copays and deductibles. $$$—if self-pay.)

k. ***Oncology nurses***: The oncology nurses administer your (IV) chemotherapy. They are not chosen by you but work at chemotherapy treatment centers. However, they are important members of your team. IV chemotherapy is essentially a low dose of poison. Your nurses must take great care, both for your sake and for his or her own. Inhaling or touching certain chemotherapy drugs can injure a nurse.

l. ***Biochemist***: This is someone usually with a Ph.D. who is doing fundamental or cutting-edge research in cancer. With a unique perspective, he or she can potentially advise you about testing using an organoid (your pancreatic cells that have been harvested alive and kept growing in a specialized laboratory) and other unconventional treatments. Unless you happen to have a relative or a friend in cancer research, consulting with a biochemist requires considerable resources ($$$+).

Emotional Support Team

a. ***Patient advocate***: Your patient advocate will form the core of your care team. This is someone who will go to most doctor visits and chemotherapy infusions with you. He or she should be someone who can raise concerns and ask questions. You might be tempted to be your own patient advocate, but you are likely to feel ill and be overwhelmed at times. Your spouse, an adult child, or a paid professional is a much better choice. Adult children often have greater computer skills than their parents, which can be very useful.

b. ***Family and friends***: You will find different ways to cope, but *people need people*. Your directions to guide your family and friends need to be practical. A general "I will do anything I can to help you" is meaningless without useful follow-up. One of the most welcome gifts can be a nutritious, home-cooked meal. There is so much else that can be done—a ride to the doctor, help with laundry, or a lunch out. You should guide your well-intended inner circle to be perceptive as to your needs and constraints, such as fatigue.[12]

Even those closest to you, the best-meaning friends and family members, may not always know what to say or do. Tell people how they can best emotionally support you. They won't be able to guess. My suggestion is to make discussing your cancer neither taboo nor compulsory.

Those less close to you are even more likely to feel the social awkwardness of not knowing what to say. You should guide them gently in the way you feel comfortable. Perhaps start by very briefly telling them about your treatment and how you are. Then guide the topic of the conversation toward them or to a common interest.

c. **Organizations / social media / nonprofits**: Faith-based organizations, local support groups, chat rooms, and Facebook are examples of where invaluable support may be available. Social media is useful because several aspects of pancreatic cancer make leaving home difficult at times. You can benefit from the general thoughts and prayers of others. Also, specific advice and empathy from those also experiencing pancreatic cancer are very valuable. Your first instinct might be to pull into your shell like a turtle, but involving others can really help you specifically and raise your spirits.

Information Management Team

a. **Data and information organizer**: Pancreatic cancer care creates a massive amount of data. There is usually someone in the family

---

12. Ibid., 146–47.

or among the patient's close friends who is good at keeping things organized. This is the perfect person for this job. This task may be broken into two categories: medical and financial. One person may organize both categories, or the categories may be managed by two people.

Medical information can be further classified as medical information about you and general information about pancreatic cancer. Some examples of the types of information that will need to be kept organized include the following:

i. Medical summary sheet
ii. History of your cancer care
iii. Laboratory results
iv. Financial records

A method for creating, storing, and updating this information follows in "Action Step Four." This is a time-consuming job. If you are in the $$ category or above, I suggest offering at least some compensation to the friend, adult child, or adult grandchild who helps. The task requires not only organizational and computer skills but also enough discipline to do updates daily or at least several times a week. For those in the $$$ and $$$$ categories, there are professionals and companies that offer patient advocacy, data management, and health-bill-review services.

b. *Information finder*: Likewise, there is often someone in your close circle who is a whiz at research. The internet and social media provide a voluminous source of data, but verifying accuracy can be a challenge. Newspapers, magazines, and books should also be read. I further recommend videos (Appendix B) to help you understand the biology of the pancreas and pancreatic cancer treatment. The American Cancer Society has a pancreatic cancer treatment summary page.[13]

The newest reliable information usually comes first in scientific journals, which are often reported by the lay press. The lay press reports about medical and scientific discoveries are usually quite accurate and easy to understand. Also, abstracts (summaries) of journal articles are often free on the internet. Generally, I suggest not reading the entire article because there will be unfamiliar words and concepts that will not relate directly to your medical care.

There are a couple of guidelines you should be aware of regarding the lay press:

- Ignore any advertising or self-promotion. Effective treatments will not need either.

- Pay attention only if the report is about new information published in a medical journal or presented at a medical conference. If it has neither of these credentials, it is probably not reliable information.

- Consider follow-up only on treatments that are already in human trials. Sadly, testing or treatment currently involving animals only will take too long to develop.

Your team should be proactive and bring ideas and questions to your oncologist. Teams can be either formal or informal. The choice of people for each role should be determined by who has the right skill set, who has available time, and who is dependable. It is alright to "fire" a member of your care team if he or she is not working out (or not compatible with the other team members) and to "hire" another.

13. American Cancer Society, "What's New in Pancreatic Cancer Research?" 2017, https://www.cancer.org/cancer/pancreatic cancer/about/new-research.html, accessed July 25, 2017.

Action Step Three: Choose or Change Your Oncologist

Physicians are licensed by the state in which they are practicing medicine. Having a medical license means that one has met the minimum qualifications to be a doctor. Board certification, in a specialty such as in oncology, is the documentation of successful advanced training and testing. The following are topics to research and questions to ask as you choose your oncologist.

First, is your oncologist's state medical license in good standing? The vast majority of physicians have unblemished medical licenses, which are called *clear and active* by many states. State boards of medicine offer an online lookup tool for doctors' licenses (see Appendix C or Campazzi.com). Look for medical-board sanctions and public complaints, which are rare. It is a yellow flag if a state has taken a disciplinary action against a physician. It is an absolute red flag if your physician is not licensed to practice medicine in the state where he or she is practicing. This is extremely rare and needs to be double-checked for an innocent explanation such as a name change from marriage.

Second, is your oncologist board certified in oncology? You can go to the American Board of Internal Medicine website (abim.org) to check this. Alternatively, you can call the American Board of Medical Specialties Certification Verification Service toll-free at 1-866-ASK-ABMS (275-2267).

Most oncologists are board certified in the medical specialty of hematology (the study of blood cells, which includes blood cancers such as leukemia and lymphoma) and oncology. The nickname for this area of medicine is *HemeOnc*. If your prospective oncologist is not board certified, more questions should be asked. It is possible to have an excellent oncologist with international training who is not eligible for US board certification. In general, the lack of board certification or lapsed board certification raises a yellow flag. Board certification lapses if an oncologist does not complete his or her maintenance of certification requirements, which include passing an examination every ten years.

The single most important role for oncologists is to prescribe and oversee the administration of chemotherapy. Chemotherapy is the most common treatment for metastatic pancreatic cancer, but it is not the only treatment. You should be alert for a potential conflict of interest with your oncologist. He or she may have a financial incentive for prescribing chemotherapy. For instance, he or she may own a chemotherapy infusion (treatment) center.

Chemotherapy may well be your best treatment, but you should have an oncologist who is willing to have an open and honest conversation with you about alternative and supplemental treatments. Ask if the oncologist or his staff is willing to do the time-consuming insurance preauthorizations needed for alternative treatments. If your oncologist is guarded or defensive about discussing alternatives, this is a yellow flag.

Common sense and instinct should play a significant role in your selection of your oncologist. If you do not feel comfortable with him or her (something just does not *feel right*), this is a reason to look for a different oncologist. If he or she does not allow generous time for questions and answers, this is a yellow flag.

A communication barrier with your oncologist is another yellow flag. Physicians are not allowed to discriminate against patients. For example, physician-patient communication for those with hearing impairment and those with limited English proficiency is addressed by Title VI of the Human Rights Act, Medicare Access and CHIP Reauthorization Act of 2015, and Section 1557 of the Affordable Care Act. State laws regarding who must provide and pay for a medical interpreter may also apply.

If English is not your first language or not your doctor's first language, there should be a medical interpreter present,[14] available by phone,[15] or available through the internet. Routinely, the medical provider, not the patient, pay for the interpreter. An interpreter is especially necessary for the first visit and for other important appointments, such as when things are not going well or when a treatment change is being considered.

It is tempting to use a relative to interpret. However, there are medical words and concepts that are difficult to explain in a second language. Also, a relative might be tempted to edit a conversation so as not to upset you, to guide treatment, or for many other reasons. I strongly recommend a professional medical translator when there is a language barrier.

If the language barrier between you and your oncologist remains despite attempts to bridge it, a red flag is raised. Communication is essential, so if there is a barrier in this area, I suggest that you pick a new

---

14. Sabriya Rice, "Hospitals Often Ignore Policies on Using Qualified Medical Interpreters," *Modern Healthcare*, August 30, 2014, http://www.modernhealthcare.com/article/20140830/MAGA-ZINE/308309945, accessed November 1, 2016.

15. Gregory Juckett and Kendra Unger, "Appropriate Use of Medical Interpreters," *American Family Physician* 90, no. 7 (October 1, 2014): 476–80, http://www.aafp.org/afp/2014/1001/p476.html, accessed November 1, 2016.

oncologist. This is true even if you sense a barrier that is too subtle to violate a law.

Given the seriousness of the discussion and the effects of normal emotions, it is a good idea to have a team member, ideally your patient advocate, take notes during your medical evaluation. While it might seem like a good idea, most doctors do not like to have audio or video recording of a medical exam. Usually, even asking puts a chill in the exam room, although there are rare physicians who are exceptions in this regard.

You may think it is a good idea to look at online physician ratings on physician review websites, but be aware that these reviews are generally of very limited value.[16] These sites usually do not verify that the patient encounter described even occurred. They can overstate negative patient experiences and do not truly reflect a doctor's competence.[17] On the other hand, reputation-management firms can put a positive spin on those doctors who deserve criticism. Take these reviews with a grain of salt.

You should have a treating oncologist who is willing to work cooperatively with other physicians and scientists. If your oncologist resists input from other professionals, this is a red flag. An interdisciplinary team is essential to give you the best possible care. At academic centers, interdisciplinary teams literally meet around a boardroom table to discuss a list of patients. This group is usually named a "Tumor Board".

You can create a virtual interdisciplinary team with specialists in many locations. While collaboration is often through e-mail, I strongly

---

16. Chandy Ellimoottil et al., "Online Physician Reviews: The Good, the Bad, and the Ugly," *Bulletin of the American College of Surgeons* 90, no. 9 (September 1, 2013), http://bulletin.facs.org/2013/09/online-physician-reviews/, accessed November 1, 2016.

17. Lacie Glover, "Are Online Physician Ratings Any Good?" *U.S. News and World Report*, December 19, 2014, http://health.usnews.com/health-news/patient-advice/articles/2014/12/19/are-online-physician-ratings-any-good, accessed November 1, 2016.

suggest that your team meet once a month on a conference call. Talking together not only improves communication but can lead to synergism (better ideas produced when a group works well together). Setting up a conference call is not technically hard to do, but coordinating schedules is difficult. If you can get more than half of your group on a call, go with that time.

You probably have already been referred or assigned to an oncologist for biopsy and initial treatment. Oncologists are very well-trained and almost universally well-motivated physicians. However, approximately three-quarters of oncologists treating pancreatic cancer are general oncologists who treat all cancers. They do not specialize in pancreatic cancer. There are oncologists, especially at major academic centers, who subspecialize in gastrointestinal cancers or even specifically in pancreatic cancer, which is one of the gastrointestinal cancers.

Ask your oncologist if he or she is a general oncologist or one who sub-specializes in the gastrointestinal tract or specifically in pancreatic cancer. I suggest a subspecialist, as he or she will have more experience and expertise with pancreatic cancer. Note that if you have pancreatic cancer, and it has spread to the liver, it is still pancreatic cancer, not liver cancer.

At any one time, you should have only one treating oncologist. It is like having one person driving the car. A key point is *you are free to change oncologists*. You can have one treating oncologist who orders medications and other consulting oncologists.

If you live in a rural area, an oncologist who does not subspecialize might be your only viable option for local treatment; however, distant specialists should give guidance should be given to your local oncologist. Receiving care locally has numerous practical advantages. Being at home is often comforting when you are ill. After the initial postdiagnosis frenzy, it is beneficial if some semblance of normal family life and career can resume.

How does one balance wanting to stay at home and getting specialty care that is only available at a distance? I lean toward the specialty care, especially soon after diagnosis. Do not be afraid to travel. Trips to seek specialty care are much like business trips, which so many people take without a second thought.

My experience with pancreatic cancer patients is that they are selfless, even to a fault. They are often hesitant to disrupt their families with trips to seek specialty care. At this moment, your family has more strength and resilience than you do. *Seek the care that you need!*

Action Step Four: Get Organized

t is essential to be highly organized. This is too big of a job to do alone, especially while sick. Have team members take charge of keeping you organized.

Sometimes, a single fact is very important. At other times, identifying a trend through a graph can guide a treatment decision. Depending on your computer literacy, you should set up a system that ranges from being largely computer based to relying on three-ring binders.

Our *paperless* society seems to generate more pieces of paper than ever before. If possible, you should scan all documents such as laboratory results, other medical records, and insurance statements. If scanned documents are labeled logically and consistently, finding and using them is so much easier. I recommend against shredding or discarding the original records for at least two years.

The most important document you need to have is an up-to-date medical summary sheet (MSS). You should take this with you whenever you seek medical care—especially if you need emergency medical treatment. You should have several preprinted copies in a folder to carry with you whenever you seek medical care. While it might be good to also have this information on a flash or thumb drive, many hospitals and health-care providers will not download your drive because of digital security concerns.

The MSS is also useful to have at more routine doctor appointments and chemotherapy infusions. In addition to your photo ID and insurance card(s), medical staff will ask for these basic facts:

1. Name of patient, contact information, insurance-policy number, social security number, and date of birth

2. Type of pancreatic cancer (e.g., adenocarcinoma) and known site(s) of metastases

3. Other patient diagnoses (e.g., diabetes and hypertension or high blood pressure)

4. Previous surgeries

5. Current medications, including dose (usually in milligrams) and number of doses per day

6. Most recent lab and imaging reports

7. CD(s) of your most recent CT scan(s)

8. Any drug allergies (nature of reaction and which year it occurred)

9. Smoking and alcohol history: Have you ever smoked? If so, for how long? How many packs per day? If you have quit, when? How many drinks per average day? Average week? Be honest, as it can only help you.

10. Name and contact information of your primary care physician and your oncologist

11. Code status: Do you want to be shocked and put on a respirator with a tube into your lungs in the case of life-threatening emergency? (You will need to confirm a "do not resuscitate" decision in the emergency department unless you have a legal document with you.)

You should keep more comprehensive information than just what is in the MSS. Whether you rely solely on your computer for information storage, have a hybrid computer-and-paper system, or keep only a paper system, you will need four basic bins:

1. A history of your treatment(s):
   b. Symptoms before diagnosis
   c. Date of diagnosis
   d. Visits to the oncologist: a summary by date of what was said and what was decided
   e. Date(s) and type(s) of all treatment(s)
   f. Any side effect(s) that you have had and which drug was thought to cause each
   g. Dates of imaging (x-rays and CT scans) as well as a copy of the reports and the physical discs; there are plastic sheets for three-ring binders to hold CDs of CT scans. If possible, get three—two extra—CDs of each CT scan to give to specialists in the future. Extra CDs should be free or available at a minimal charge ($)

2. Whatever you are learning about pancreatic cancer, always make a note on the document stating where you found the information, whether it was from a person, a book, a website, or a video, and keep this information. For example, note the URL and time into a

video where helpful information is found. Types of information you should keep notes about include the following:

a. New treatments
b. Alternative treatments
c. Ways to minimize side effects
d. Diets
e. Supplements

3. Keep all your laboratory reports and test results in one place and in chronological order. If you have blood drawn in your oncologist's office and you develop a fever on a Saturday night, for example, it will help the emergency department staff if you can bring laboratory results with you. Ideally, the hospital could access these results directly, but that is not always the case. For those familiar with Excel (a spreadsheet program), I have a template for recording lab values over time available for download on my website, Campazzi.com.

4. You will probably receive a maddening number of "explanation of benefits" statements and other financial statements from your doctors—even more so if you receive hospital services. There are often redundant mailings. My suggestions to manage them are:

a. After scanning, keep all paperwork together—a three-ring binder is best for this, but labeled cardboard boxes will also work.
b. Keep your paperwork in order by date of service, not by the date of the invoice.
c. Clip seemingly redundant things together with a paper clip, but do not throw out anything for at least a couple of years.

Action Step Five: Get A Pathology Second Opinion

A pathology slide is a single layer of your cells on a glass slide. Your cells are stained with various chemicals so that they can be seen clearly under a microscope. Images of slides can be digitized for computer-assisted evaluation. Doctors who read (examine) these slides are pathologists. Their work is very important to you. The pathologist makes the final and definitive diagnosis of pancreatic cancer while the radiologist determines if it has metastasized (spread to other parts of the body).

The pathologist diagnoses the type of pancreatic cancer you have. Adenocarcinoma accounts for 95 percent of pancreatic cancer.[18] Neuroendocrine tumors make up most of the other 5 percent.[19] The pathologist also gives more in-depth technical information to your oncologist, such as the aggressiveness and subtype of your cancer cells.

---

18. American Cancer Society, "What Is Pancreatic Cancer?," http://www.cancer.org/cancer/pancreatic-cancer/detailedguide/pancreatic cancer-what-is-pancreatic cancer, Last Modified May 31, 2016, accessed November 1, 2016.

19. Ibid.

While *I strongly recommend a pathology second opinion for everyone*, a pathology second opinion is *a must for patients with islet cell or neuroendocrine tumors*. These rare tumors can be malignant or nonmalignant and of several subtypes. The differences between the different types are usually subtle. For all, engaging a pathologist with specific expertise in pancreatic cancer is essential. The effectiveness of your treatment depends on an accurate diagnosis by your pathologist.

The information from your pathologist is the basis for your treatment. If your pathology is incorrectly interpreted, virtually everything that follows will be wrong, and it could even be harmful to you. Consequently, the opinion of the pathologist who originally diagnosed your cancer at your local hospital needs to be double-checked.

You can easily locate an academic medical center to which your pathology slides can be sent. Options can be found through an internet search of the phrase *pathology second opinion*. The cost for a second opinion on your pathology is likely to be about $250 but can be higher if further tests are needed. Most of the time, your original pathologist will be right; however, it is imperative to find an incorrect diagnosis early. Even finding a small difference in subtype can improve your treatment outcome.

Action Step Six: Get An Oncology Second Opinion(s)

R emember, the wisest expert knows only a fraction of what there is to know. Having pancreatic cancer forces you to think outside the box because current treatment has limited benefits and severe side effects. Why would you rely solely on the expertise of your oncologist?

Whenever possible and if your resources allow it, I suggest traveling to an academic medical center to meet in person with an oncologist who subspecializes in pancreatic cancer and get a second opinion. Do not wait to make the appointment until you have the second pathology reading because you do not have that much time. The consulting oncologist can review the pathology results either before or after you see him or her.

Doctors at major cancer centers can help you best by examining you in person and talking with you face-to-face. Many community oncologists treat all cancers so they will not have the in-depth expertise of a subspecialist. With some insurances, seeing a specialist at a cancer center has no more out-of-pocket cost than seeing a local oncologist.

According to Johns Hopkins Medicine,

Having a list of questions prepared in advance is useful for making the time you have with the doctor as efficient and helpful as possible. Here is a list to help you get started:

1. What type of pancreatic cancer do I have?

2. What stage of disease do you believe I have based on what you know from my clinical examination, x-rays, pathology, and tests done so far?

3. Can my cancer be taken out with surgery, and if so, by what type of pancreatic surgery?

4. Did the pathology team confirm the accuracy of the biopsy results?

5. How soon would my surgery be scheduled?

6. What educational information do you offer to prepare me for surgery and what to expect?

7. Who will be my contact here for questions I may have?

8. Do you have educational materials for other family members, like my children?

9. How many pancreatic surgeries do you perform a year?

10. How long have you been in practice doing pancreatic surgeries?

11. Who else will be involved in my care, and when will I meet those persons?

12. Will I need more therapy (chemotherapy and/or radiation therapy) after surgery? How soon after surgery?

13. How often will I need to see you after my surgery for ongoing evaluation?

14. Are there clinical trials that you recommend for me to consider at this point?

15. Who will be coordinating my care? Do you have a patient navigator?

16. How are future appointments arranged for me, and when do these happen?[20]

If you cannot make the trip to a major treatment center, there is another option that is nearly as good. Many cancer centers offer a *chart review*. They will read your medical records and often will also directly look at your diagnostic images (x-rays and CT scans). Their recommendations can change your treatment and thus your life. For those in the $ and $$ categories, I would consider this expenditure of about $1,000, which may not be covered by your health insurance. To find a doctor who can do this for you, do an internet search for the term *remote second opinion cancer*. I recommend using academic medical centers with large oncology departments.

There is an adage that goes something like, if you go to a shoe store, they will tell you that you need a new pair of shoes. If you go to a bar, they will ask, "Need a brew?". Take the opportunity to ask the oncologist offering a second opinion about treatments that your treating oncologist may not offer. Do not assume that your treating oncologist can offer all

---

20. Nita Ahuja and JoAnn Coleman, *Patient's Guide to Pancreatic Cancer*, (Burlington, MA: Jones and Bartlett Learning, 2012), 35–37, www.jblearning.com, reprinted with permission.

possible treatments or that he or she will suggest a treatment that he or she does not offer. An example is low-dose chemotherapy. As part of your second opinion, you should also ask about any new treatments showing great promise that you find by searching the internet, using Google Alerts, and having discussions with your care team.

Action Step Seven: Consider An
Interventional Radiology Opinion

B efore deciding on a course of treatment, you also might want to consider consulting with an interventional radiologist. For instance, the
Y-90 procedure might be an option. Intra-arterial yttrium-90 radioembolization is a procedure in which extremely tiny (five times the size
of a red blood cell) radioactive beads are placed in liver metastases from
pancreatic cancer. "Radioembolization is a *palliative*, not a curative, treatment. Patients benefit by having their lives extended while experiencing
milder and fewer side effects compared to chemotherapy. For instance, you
could avoid severe fatigue that can last for seven to ten days after some
chemotherapy."[21]

It is unusual to seek this consultation early in the course of treatment.
The mainstays of treatment are, first, chemotherapy and, second, conventional radiation therapy. This approach is usually not considered unless the
patient has failed at least two other treatments.

---

21. "Y-90 Liver Cancer-Busting Treatment: Safe, Fast, Extends Life, Study Finds," *Science Daily*, March 28,
2011. https://www.sciencedaily.com/releases/2011/03/110328092409.htm, accessed November 1, 2016.

I believe that patients should make informed choices with the knowledge of all options. While the vast majority of patients should accept the standard-of-care treatments, avoiding treatment side effects is the first priority of some patients. It is important to realize that after a Y-90 procedure, you would still have all the symptoms that stem directly from the pancreatic cancer in your pancreas but probably only few and mild symptoms from this alternative treatment. Still, for those with metastatic pancreatic cancer in the liver, Y-90 can minimize symptoms from liver metastases and extend life, as the most common cause of death from pancreatic cancer is liver failure.[22]

---

22. Ibid.

Action Step Eight: Consider A Second Biopsy For An Organoid

An organoid is a three-dimensional growth of your cells (but it doesn't resemble a pancreas) grown in a laboratory and can be tested against a very large number of different drugs and drug combinations. One decision you should make before starting treatment is whether you wish to have your live tumor cells harvested to grow in an organoid. *The best results are obtained with cells that have never been exposed to chemotherapy in your body.*

Through this process, hundreds of chemotherapeutic and other drugs can be tested for effectiveness with a technique called high-throughput analysis. These drugs can be further tested in thousands of combinations.

Organoid testing is not currently widely available, but I believe it potentially offers very significant benefits. It is *designed to find drugs that kill your tumor cells.* Most of these medications are currently licensed in the United States, sometimes to treat other diseases.

For instance, a recent Johns Hopkins study[23] found that a drug, tocilizumab, blocks cancer metastasis in mice. This drug is already FDA approved and

23. Hasini Jayatilaka et al., "Synergistic IL-6 and IL-8 Paracrine Signalling Pathway Infers a Strategy to Inhibit Tumour Cell Migration," *Nature Communications* 8 (2017): 15584, DOI:10.1038/ncomms15584.

in use to treat rheumatoid arthritis. A doctor could immediately prescribe it for what is called an *off-label* use if organoid testing suggested it for you.

Another example is Antabuse (disulfiram), which has been used for a long time to treat alcoholics. In early testing of organoids, Antabuse killed or markedly slowed the growth of pancreatic cancer cells for many patients. Again, since it is already available, doctors can prescribe this medication. The caveat is that a patient cannot drink even a sip of alcohol while taking Antabuse, as it would cause severe nausea and vomiting.

Growing organoids requires harvesting live tumor cells and handling them specially until they reach the laboratory. This requires a second biopsy, which is an invasive procedure. Another challenge of organoids is the cost, which is in the $$$ range and not covered by insurance. Consider looking for clinical trials involving organoids ($) and discussing this option with your oncologist.

Those with metastases in their liver have one advantage over those with cancer only in the pancreas. It is technically easier to biopsy metastases, especially in the liver than to biopsy cancer in the pancreas. Since the cells in the metastatic tumors are metastatic cancer cells from your pancreas, they are the same as the ones in your primary tumor. The more live cells you can harvest, the faster you can grow and test an organoid, so a biopsy of liver metastases can be advantageous.

To obtain a sufficient volume of cells, you will need a minimally invasive surgical procedure. Under anesthesia, a catheter is guided either through the skin or through your jugular vein to the site of your metastases. This should be done by a physician with experience in this procedure. The liver has high volume blood flow, so the procedure must be done properly to avoid internal bleeding afterward.

A simple blood draw called a liquid biopsy is an alternative to a surgical biopsy. Some patients are on blood thinners for the treatment of other diseases or have a genetic bleeding tendency. For them, a liquid biopsy is likely a better alternative. Very few tumor cells circulate in the blood of those with pancreatic cancer. Some of these can be collected with a liquid biopsy. The downside of this procedure is that it harvests so little tumor material. Running tests is technically challenging but possible when the number of tumor cells available is limited, and organoids starting from only a few cells take a long time to grow to a size sufficient for testing.

The cells in an organoid can take months to grow. While it is theoretically possible to grow enough cells for testing in two weeks, this goal is not routinely obtained. More information is available in a short video from the Sanger Institute. I recommend that you watch, at least, the first two minutes of their video.[24] Results from organoid testing will probably not be available in time to guide your first choice of chemotherapy, but the information can be very valuable at about the two-month mark when a change in medications is often needed.

Organoids are a great tool but one that has yet to be perfected or offered commercially. As of the writing of this book, you would have to find and enroll in a clinical trial to take advantage of this technology. Perhaps by the time you are reading this book, however, organoids and high-throughput testing will be available commercially.

Dr. David Tuveson of Cold Spring Harbor Laboratories and Dr. Hans Clevers of the Dutch Science Foundation pioneered this work. The Lustgarten Foundation is a sponsor of research about pancreatic tumor organoids. The Scripps Research Institute has led the way with high-throughput testing research. You will need to do an internet search on the term *pancreatic cancer organoid clinical research* to find where studies are being conducted.

---

24. Sanger Institute, "Organoids: Cancer in 3D," May 7, 2015, https://www.youtube.com/watch?v=DH9m-4bRYOc, accessed November 1, 2016.

Action Step Nine: Consider Genetic Analysis, Counseling, And Treatment

Acquired and inherited genetic defects are what cause pancreatic cancer. Thus, learning about these defects is the key to transforming pancreatic cancer from a deadly disease to a chronic disease that is manageable and does not kill you. Eventually, genetics will enable us to accurately predict who will get pancreatic cancer and may even provide a cure. We will then be able to intervene to prevent the disease or at least monitor patients closely (a process called surveillance) for early signs of the disease and then treat it effectively.

Three reasons for having genetic studies ($$–$$$) are as follows:

1. **To assess medicines for effectiveness in you**: Only 10 to 15 percent of patients will have a genetic defect in their tumor that is matched to an effective treatment.[25] Please note that this percentage is growing. Knowing which drugs will work for an individual patient is a huge advantage in his or her care. It is a red flag if your

---

25. Sol Goldman Pancreatic Cancer Research Center, "Is Pancreatic Cancer Hereditary?," http://pathology.jhu.edu/pc/basicheredity.php?area=ba, accessed November 1, 2016.

oncologist advises against getting genetic studies done because "we won't know what to do with the results."

Sequencing the entire tumor genome produces lots of data, only some of which is actionable information. However, genetic analysis is quickly becoming more informative. For instance, if breast cancer has an amplification of the HER2 gene, drugs like trastuzumab can be considered. If colon cancer shows with a normal KRAS gene, consideration should be given to erlotinib. *And if your cancer—regardless of its type (including pancreatic cancer), has a defective DNA-mismatch-repair system, consideration should be given to Keytruda.*[26] *If you are going to get only one supplemental test, get the test for a defective DNA-mismatch-repair system/microsatellite instability.*

Keytruda is an FDA-approved drug that your oncologist can prescribe. Keytruda's FDA approval was recently broadened because Keytruda is effective in treating multiple types of cancer that have certain specific characteristics.[27]

2. **To determine whether your cancer is hereditary or inheritable**: Genetic testing can tell you if you are among those who have a gene that predisposes them to pancreatic cancer. Approximately 10 percent of pancreatic cancers are inherited.

The likelihood that you have an inheritable form of pancreatic cancer is higher if one of your first-degree relatives (parents, siblings, or children) has previously been diagnosed with pancreatic cancer. Regardless, you should speak with a genetic counselor to assess your family's risk. Pancreatic cancer can be related to a family

---

26. Dr. Bert Vogelstein, e-mail message to author, June 24, 2017.

27. Emily Netburn, "New Cancer Drug Defeats Multiple Tumors," *Newsmax* June 16, 2017, http://www. newsmax.com/Health/Cancer/keytruda-immunotherapy-cancer-breakthrough/2017/06/16/id/796473/.

history of melanoma, other gastrointestinal cancers (colon cancer, for example), and BRCA 1 and 2, which are genes closely related to breast cancer.

Unfortunately, knowing of a familial risk currently offers few practical options, as no screening test for pancreatic cancer is available. This is a list of imperfect ways of detection:

a. CA 19-9 is a sugar found on the surface of pancreatic tumors. It circulates in your blood, and detection requires only a routine blood draw. In general, levels of CA 19-9 go up and down with the effectiveness of treatment. However, CA 19-9 cannot be reliably used for looking for pancreatic cancer. Usually, the level of CA 19-9 does not increase until a tumor is large. Furthermore, there are other reasons that CA 19-9 levels can increase besides pancreatic cancer.

b. A CT scan is the best imaging technique for the initial diagnosis of pancreatic cancer. When done repetitively, the cumulative radiation exposure from CTs poses health risks.

c. Endoscopic ultrasounds arguably produce the best images of early pancreatic cancer. Requiring a tube down your esophagus into your stomach, it is invasive and requires anesthesia, and someone experienced in viewing the pancreas is necessary for a reliable result. Therefore, it is quite costly and best done at an academic medical center that specializes in pancreatic cancer.[28]

d. Magnetic resonance cholangiopancreatography (MRCP) is an MRI that is done after an IV dye is given to you. It has proven to successfully reveal a developing pancreatic cancer only when the person has the CDKN2A mutation, one of the many possible genetic defects. MRCP has not been proven (a high

---

28. Hiroyoshi Furukawa, "Diagnostic Clues for Early Pancreatic Cancer," *Japanese Journal of Clinical Oncology* 32, no. 10 (2002): 391–92.

standard) to be a good screening test in other circumstances, although it offers potential.

e. Liquid biopsy is a technology in early development that uses a routine peripheral blood draw to find a tiny trace of tumor DNA (being developed commercially in the United States) or RNA (undergoing testing in Japan[29]) in the circulating blood. This gives the best hope for the future of early diagnosis leading to early and successful treatment. Check if liquid biopsies for pancreatic cancer are available by the time you are reading this book.

If your pancreatic cancer is not hereditary, you are among the 90 percent whose pancreatic cancer is randomly acquired. If you have randomly acquired cancer, your DNA was damaged at some point—probably multiple times—during your lifetime, leading to cancer formation.

3. **To understand your tumor**: Today, genetic research is shifting into high gear. It cost $3 billion and took thirteen years to first sequence the entire human genome in 2003. For about $1,000 and in just a few days, your tumor-cell genome can now be sequenced ($$). A DNA sequencing generates voluminous data, but much of it is labeled *variant of unknown significance*. This term means that a gene is abnormal, but with current knowledge and technology, the result does not provide any useful information.

If you want to take genetic testing even further, a more expensive test called RNA sequencing will tell you which of the genes in your tumor cells are active. Since this data is not *yet* useful for either treatment or prevention, I recommend these tests for only those in the $$$ and $$$$ categories.

---

29. *The Japan News*, "New Blood Test Can Check for 13 Types of Cancers," July 24, 2017, http://www.the-japan-news.com/news/article/0003837884.

Genetics-based treatment is the goal, as it would treat the root cause of pancreatic cancer: genetic defects. The basic technique is to insert a normal human gene into a non-harmful virus and then infect the patient with the virus. Viruses work by inserting themselves into human DNA thus carrying the needed normal gene into millions of cells in the body. This complex treatment is being studied (and is not yet approved) for several diseases with increasing success.

While not directly relevant to pancreatic cancer, in July 2017, an FDA panel unanimously recommended that the agency approve the first-ever treatment that genetically alters patients' cells to treat leukemia. A study of sixty-three patients supported the Novartis treatment. Notably, Emily Whitehead was six years old in 2012 when she did not respond to conventional treatment. A blood sample from her was sent to a laboratory, and a cancer-fighting gene was inserted using a modified/noninfectious HIV virus. The blood was then reinfused into her. After severe side-effects for two weeks, she was apparently cured. She testified before the FDA on behalf of the treatment five years after it saved her life.[30] It is hoped that a similar combination of genetic therapy and immunotherapy will be available for pancreatic cancer in the future.

---

30. Denise Grady, "F.D.A. Panel Recommends Approval for Gene-Altering Leukemia Treatment," *The New York Times*, July 12, 2017, https://www.nytimes.com/2017/07/12/health/fda-novartis-leukemia-gene-medicine.html.

Action Step Ten: Consider Immune System–Based Treatments

Walt Disney had a saying: "Plus it."

One way to create *chemotherapy plus* is to add immune-based treatment. Immunotherapy also called biologic therapy, is a type of cancer treatment that boosts the body's natural defenses to fight cancer. It uses substances made by the body or in a laboratory to improve or restore immune-system function. Immunotherapy may work in these ways:

- Stopping or slowing the growth of cancer cells

- Stopping cancer from spreading to other parts of the body

- Helping the immune system better destroy cancer cells

There are several types of immunotherapy, including those listed here:

- Monoclonal antibodies

- Nonspecific immunotherapies

- Oncolytic virus therapy

- T-cell therapy

- Cancer vaccines[31]

Ideally, immunotherapy has the added benefit of circulating throughout the body, killing microscopic metastases. It is an area of active study, generally comes with few side effects, and usually does not interfere with chemotherapy. The downside is that while virtually every immune-based approach sounds great, in theory, many have failed to demonstrate any effect in large-scale trials.

The immune system has two basic components. The T-cell is a type of white blood cell circulating in your blood. T-cells can be considered *soldier cells* because they can directly kill cancer cells. The second component is antibodies, which are proteins that circulate in the blood like cruise missiles. These proteins specifically target one thing that can harm the body. For instance, immunizations such as the flu shot cause the body to make antibodies to kill flu viruses if they infect you.

These are some examples of cancer immunotherapy:

1. **Vaccines**: Unlike most vaccines, which are given to prevent disease, there are vaccines are designed to treat cancer. The FDA has approved vaccines for prostate cancer and melanoma. They stimulate the immune system to fight tumors. Vaccines to fight pancreatic cancer are in clinical trials as of the summer of 2017. They tend

---

31. Cancer.Net Editorial Board, ed., "Understanding Immunotherapy," April 2017, http://www.cancer.net/navigating-cancer-care/how-cancer-treated/immunotherapy-and-vaccines/understanding-immunotherapy, accessed June 22, 2017, reprinted with permission.

to produce fewer and less severe side effects than chemotherapy. Pancreatic cancer vaccines have not proven to be very effective but still hold promise for future success.

2. **Checkpoint inhibitors**: The body's immune system must be able to tell friend from foe. Part of the way this is accomplished is through the proteins on the surface of normal cells that function as ID badges. The immune system does not attack cells with the appropriate cell-surface markers. Tumor cells can produce or even overproduce proteins that inhibit your immune system. Checkpoint inhibition overcomes this defense, which otherwise protects your cancer. This approach is under study but has yet to be approved for pancreatic cancer in the United States.

Keytruda and Yervoy are checkpoint inhibitors that have been approved for melanoma. Doctors can legally and ethically use a drug approved for one disease to treat another. Again, this is called off-label use. Usually, special laboratory testing is needed to see if these medications will likely work for you.

3. **Personalized medicine**: In general, personalized medicine is treatment tailored specifically to your results from a variety of scientific testing. For example, there are experimental techniques in which your white blood cells are harvested from an ordinary blood draw. A subset that is most likely to attack your tumor is selected and grown manyfold in the laboratory. These cells are then injected back into you to attack your tumor.

In addition to the United States, Germany is leading the way in immunotherapy. Denmark, England, Israel, and Korea are also actively researching the immune system and different types of cancer. There is definitely great work being done outside the United States. As of summer 2017, immunotherapy for pancreatic cancer is a work in progress.

Action Step Eleven: Consider A Radiation Oncologist's Opinion

Radiation oncology is not usually the first-line treatment of metastatic pancreatic cancer; chemotherapy is. Chemotherapy is carried throughout your body in your bloodstream. It can kill tiny metastases too small to see on your CT scan. Radiation therapy (RT) on the other hand, kills cancer only where it is precisely aimed.

RT has some of the same limitations as surgery. As seen in earlier images, the pancreas is deep in the center of your body. It is surrounded by the stomach, the bowel, and major blood vessels. Like the surgeon's scalpel, RT can inadvertently damage these important parts of the body.

The depth of the pancreas in the body causes technical challenges, as the radiation must pass through normal tissue without causing damage. The basis of RT is to aim radiation beams from several different directions, with the focal point of the beams being your cancer mass. Each of the beams is weak enough that it should not damage normal tissue, but at the intersection of the beams, there is enough radiation to kill the tumor cells. RT can also be used to shrink the largest cancer masses to avoid blockage of the pancreatic or bile ducts.

RT is a potential option for those wishing to substitute the similar but often milder side effects of RT for the side effects of chemotherapy. While RT also causes loss of appetite, diarrhea, nausea, and fatigue, these side effects are generally less severe than those of chemotherapy drugs.

Radiation therapy uses x-rays, and other types of energy focused on your tumor to kill cells. RT comes in several varieties:

1. **Conventional external-beam RT**: This treatment is given in relatively low doses daily for about five weeks, and the idea is to allow surrounding tissue to recover between treatments and thus minimize collateral damage and side effects.

2. **High-dose RT (stereotactic)**: This is also called "radiosurgery" and "cybersurgery." It is given in four to six sessions for maximized effect and for patient convenience. With this more aggressive approach, the side effects listed above are more likely and more severe.

3. **Intensity-modulated and image-guided RT:** These are advanced technologies that increase the precision of RT and are only available at some centers, generally academic and specialized centers. The advantage of this type of treatment is dependent on the details of your pancreatic cancer.

4. **Brachytherapy:**
   a. *Temporary*: A probe inserted near or into your tumor administers a large dose of radiation for a few minutes.
   b. *Permanent*: Metallic seeds that emit a low dose of radiation over many days are placed directly in your cancer mass. This is often used to treat large liver metastases. The previously discussed Y-90 procedure is an example of brachytherapy.

You can ask either your primary care physician or your oncologist for a radiation-oncologist recommendation or go the U.S. News & World Report website.[32] Insurance coverage varies widely, but there is a possibility that your radiation oncology consult will not be covered since it is not considered first-line treatment ($$). I recommend you see a radiation oncologist before starting chemotherapy for the following reasons:

1. There might be something unique about your cancer that would make RT the better option.

2. There might have been advances in RT since this book was written.

3. Radiation oncologists assess pancreatic cancer from a different perspective than medical oncologists do. If no RT can be offered, something else of value for your treatment might be recommended by your radiation oncologist.

---

32. "Find Radiation Oncologists," *U.S. News & World Report*, Last Modified 2017, http://health.usnews.com/doctors/location-index/radiation-oncologists, accessed July 25, 2017.

Action Step Twelve: Choose Your Initial Treatment

No matter what profession you are in, a person without relevant experience cannot obtain a fraction of your expertise through an afternoon of Googling. Think of the eager real-estate shopper who finds a house in a good school district at 25 percent less per square footage than comparable houses. It looks just as great on a walk through. Then the experienced real-estate agent steps in and reveals that the wind is not from the north today. If it were, there would be a considerable odor from the landfill. This is why the price seems low.

By reading this book and other material, I hope you become an informed consumer/patient, but please do not consider yourself an instant expert. You need to depend heavily on your treating oncologist to guide the important decision of what your initial treatment should be. Since pancreatic cancer generally affects patients in their fifties, sixties, and seventies, your oncologist will recommend treatment bearing in mind your overall health, including any medications you regularly take.

For many, starting treatment with chemotherapy will be your only viable option. However, this choice should be a truly informed decision. This table from Texas Oncology summarizes the limited results expected from traditional chemotherapy:

Table 1: Results from seven trials that evaluated different chemotherapy regimens in the treatment of advanced pancreatic cancer[33]

	Response rate	One-year survival	Overall survival
Gemzar / Platinol (cisplatin)	26%	NA***	7.5 months
Gemzar / Camptosar (irinotecan)	32%	27%	9 months
Gemzar / Alimta (pemetrexed)	15%	30%	6.5 months
Gemzar / Eloxatin (oxaliplatin)	30* or 31%**	26* or 47%**	NA***
Gemzar / 5FU / Platinol / Ellence (epirubicin)	58%	NA***	11 months
Taxotere (docetaxel) / Doxil (doxorubicin)	30%	33%	10 months
Gemzar / Taxotere / Xeloda (capecitabine)	47%	NA***	NA***

*patients with locally advanced disease (IVA)
**patients with metastatic disease (IVB)
***not measured in this trial

Chemotherapy drugs are essentially poisons that target the most rapidly dividing cells. Chemotherapy circulates throughout your entire body, which is both good and bad. It can treat tiny metastases that are too small to detect.

---

33. Texas Oncology, Last Modified 2017, https://www.texasoncology.com/types-of-cancer/pancreatic cancer/stage-iv-pancreatic cancer/, accessed May 30, 2017, reprinted with permission.

However, cancer cells are not the only rapidly dividing cells in the body. In the adult body, most cells do not divide or grow. There are significant exceptions, such as bone-marrow cells, which produce new red blood cells; hair cells; and the cells lining the gastrointestinal tract all the way from the mucosa of the mouth through the colon. Since chemotherapy drugs are nonspecific, powerful, and toxic, they also affect the normal fast-growing cells listed above.

Great care must be taken with chemotherapy. This is a primary focus of the oncologist's work. He or she must provide medical care that meets the definition of standard of care, which is determined by state (not federal) law. Standard of care is essentially what the average specialty physician would do under similar circumstances.[34]

More than one treatment can be within the standard of care. While doctors often worry about being sued for malpractice, the legal definition of standard of care certainly allows for some discretion or flexibility on the part of the doctor. This is termed "second school of thought"[35] or "respected minority opinion."[36] Treatment can and should be tailored to the specifics of your medical condition and to your input, if reasoned and informed.

Chemotherapy is the standard of care for most cases of metastatic pancreatic cancer as of summer 2017 and is associated with limited but life-lengthening results. The standard of care may not be the best care, as new treatments are constantly under development. Rather, the standard is also defined as the "customary practice of average

---

34. David Goguen, "What is the Medical Standard of Care? Medical Malpractice Lawsuits Stem from a Medical Professional's Deviation from This Legal Obligation That They Owe Their Patients," http://www.alllaw.com/articles/nolo/medical-malpractice/standard-of-care.html, accessed May 30, 2017.

35. Ibid.

36. Ibid.

physicians"[37]using therapies (drugs and other types of treatment) approved by the US Food and Drug Administration. For a therapy to become the new standard of care, it would have to meet the strict criteria of being *proven better* than the treatment deemed to be the previous standard of care.

Again, for most, I suggest *chemotherapy plus*, meaning traditional care plus additional treatments or supplements. What to choose for the *plus* is a decision you should make with the help of a well-qualified and open-minded oncologist and the team you have supporting you. Together you should review all treatment options. As you choose what to add to your standard of care, use these guiding principles:

1. **Make sure that you are doing no harm.** For instance, there is the real concern that mega-high-dose vitamin C (fifty grams IV) decreases chemotherapy side effects by substantially inactivating it.

2. **Make no unforced errors.** This is a tennis term I use to say that you should avoid simple mistakes like not understanding the directions for taking a medicine or unintentionally missing a medical appointment. Double-check everything that you can. Use reminders for medications and upcoming appointments. Allow your team members to help you wherever possible. There is a lot that is out of your control about this disease. Focus on the aspects you can positively affect.

3. **Have some scientific evidence, even if it's not conclusive.** This will be important to let you make a decision regarding treatment. Again, scientific evidence is found in medical journals and at medical conferences. The lay press referring to these is the key to finding information.

---

37. Ibid.

4. **Use common sense.** This is a simple phrase that most people intuitively understand. Despite the fear and other emotions that you are likely feeling, you need to take a moment to reflect and use your best judgment before making any major decisions.

What if you decide against chemotherapy? Since chemotherapy is the only treatment with the proven capability to extend your life by a few, several, or even many months, the medical community guides you to take it. Enrolling in a clinical trial is risky because, by definition, the effectiveness of new medications and nondrug treatments is not known.

Johns Hopkins Medicine suggests, "a list of questions that you should consider asking to help guide you in decision making and fact-finding about clinical trials":

- What is the purpose of the study?

- How many people will be included in the study?

- What does the study involve? What kind of tests and treatment will I have?

- How are treatments given and what side effects might I expect?

- What are the risks and benefits of each protocol?

- What alternatives do I have to participating in the study?

- How long will the study last?

- What type of long-term follow-up care is provided for those who participate?

- Will I incur any costs? Will my insurance company pay for part of this?

- When will the results be known?"[38]

Trials are governed by institutional review boards, well-intended ethics committees composed of scientists and nonscientists. Their guidance can seem a little heavy-handed. For instance, often to participate in a clinical trial, you must have *failed* (meaning treatment did not work or stopped working) two chemotherapy regimens (one or a combination of drugs).

You may have heard that clinical trials in other countries, such as Australia, are easier to participate in. It would be very unlikely but not impossible that this would be a good idea for you. Many drugs have seemed highly effective in early trials only to be ineffective or harmful in large trials. If you are interested in receiving care internationally, which is called *medical tourism*, discuss this at length with your treating and consulting oncologists. Do not let a sense of desperation lead you to chase rainbows.

In addition to chemotherapy medications, there are additional medications with some, but not conclusive, evidence that they could help control pancreatic cancer. They are as follows:

1. **Disulfiram (Antabuse)**: A surprising finding from testing pancreatic tumor organoids is that disulfiram seems to slow tumor-cell growth and make several chemotherapy drugs more effective. Disulfiram is used to treat alcoholics because it causes severe nausea and vomiting if any alcohol is ingested. This is a preliminary finding and is under further study. You could ask your oncologist if he or she recommends it.

---

38. Ahuja, Nita and JoAnn Coleman, *Patient's Guide to Pancreatic Cancer*, (2012: Jones and Bartlett Learning, Burlington, MA.): 56. www.jblearning.com Reprinted with permission.

2. **Hyaluronidase (brand name Halozyme)**: It achieved fast-track FDA approval for treatment of metastatic pancreatic cancer in September 2014. This medicine can be added to your chemotherapy to help break down the net of fiber (back cover) that grows with your tumor cells, seemingly to protect them from your immune system and chemotherapy. This drug acts like a machete does in the jungle to clear a path for a variety of treatments to access your pancreatic cancer cells.

3. **Metformin**: There is conflicting evidence about the use of this medication usually prescribed for mild diabetes. Pancreatic cancer can cause diabetes, but the question is whether to add metformin to your pancreatic cancer treatment if you have not developed diabetes, as some studies do suggest a benefit. Since the evidence is mixed, discuss this idea with your oncologist.

   Metformin is an old and thus well-studied medication that generally has few side effects. My reading of these studies is that while it may or may not be helpful in fighting cancer, it seems to do no harm.

4. **Keytruda**: Keytruda is the drug President Carter took for melanoma that had metastasized to his brain. According to publicly available information, he has achieved full remission.

   If your genetic testing reveals DNA-repair-pathway defects or "microsatellite instability," consideration should be given to Keytruda or other similar medicines.[39] Let me reiterate that you should be tested (just a tube of blood is needed) for *a defective*

---

39. Pancreatic Action Network, "Unprecedented Drug Approval Can Benefit Pancreatic Cancer Patients," Last Modified May 24, 2017, https://www.pancan.org/news/unprecedented-drug-approval-can-benefit-pancreatic-cancer-patients/, accessed July 25, 2017.

DNA-mismatch-repair system because it can change your treatment to a drug that could quite possibly be more effective ($$).

5. **Medicines not licensed in the United States**: High-speed and high-volume throughput testing is currently being done on an experimental basis at Scripps Florida. In the laboratory, they can test *your* pancreatic cancer cells with 3,200 drugs and drug combinations. Included in Scripps testing are all medications used to fight pancreatic cancer worldwide. Some of these medications are not licensed for use in the United States, some for safety reasons and others for commercial reasons. While I believe that the most effective chemotherapy medications are used and licensed in the United States, laboratory testing including drugs used only in foreign countries is wise. While the odds of finding an effective drug licensed only outside the United States are low, they are not zero ($$$–$$$$).

   If a medication used only abroad were to be found highly effective for you, there could be creative options, including travel, to discuss with your oncologist. Again, you would need to research extensively before considering these.

Finally, discussion and consideration should be given to the addition of genetic therapy, immune-based therapy, and interventional radiology as previously discussed.

Action Step Thirteen: Engage Pain Management And Nursing

Pancreatic cancer can be very painful. Your pain can be effectively managed by narcotic medication, which is best to have prescribed by an expert, a palliative medicine doctor. Sometimes a time-released drug such as fentanyl (a strong medication in the opioid class) is given through a small patch attached to your skin. This would need to be changed only every three days. An opiate patch often causes less nausea and vomiting than pills.

The ideal team in the home includes both nurses and family. On days when you have fever, nausea, pain, or diarrhea, assistance from a nurse will be most welcome. You probably won't want to be alone, yet you might not want to impose these symptoms on a family member, either. During hours or days when you are feeling well, you will most likely want to spend time with family and friends.

Professional home nurses can be very valuable in helping you through side effects from both your cancer and its treatment. If it is affordable, having a nurse is beneficial because a nurse knows how to make patients more comfortable during difficult times. The nurses also know when to be in touch with the physician. They can anticipate and often prevent discomfort.

Nursing aides can also be effective by offering measures to help relieve side effects from medications. Unlike nurses, nursing aides cannot give medicines to patients. Patients or their families must know which medication is needed, what the dosage is, and when it must be given.

The states license healthcare providers, including nurses. Therefore, there are differences in licensure requirements and designations. Across most states, these are the different levels of nurses who provide in-home care:

1. **Registered nurses (RNs) ($$$$)**: RNs have received two to four years of advanced education and have passed an exam to be licensed by the state. With physician supervision, they direct and provide care in hospitals, homes, nursing homes, and schools.

2. **Licensed practical nurses (LPNs) or licensed vocational nurses (title used in California and Texas) ($$$+)**: LNPs have a minimum of one year of training after graduating from high school or the equivalent. LPNs work under the direction of doctors or RNs.

3. **Certified Nursing Assistants ($$+)**: Certified Nursing Assistants have a minimum of six weeks of instruction and have passed an examination. They are not technically considered nurses, although they can be very helpful. They are often hired for overnight shifts.

4. **Nursing assistants ($$)**: Nursing assistants have not passed a state examination or completed a state-required examination.

In-home nursing services should be individually tailored. The assumption that there is no need for a nurse or an aide while you sleep at night may not be true. Some patients have night sweats that necessitate sponge baths and multiple changes of sleepwear. The following assumes 24-7 care, but the recommendations can be adjusted for your needs and budgets:

1. **Nursing agencies**: The easiest way to hire nurses is through a nursing agency. Agencies attempt to select the best nurses, do background checks, and supervise their nurses. They recruit, schedule, and pay nurses. An additional 50 percent to 100 percent above what the nurse receives is charged for these services. A registered nurse hired through an agency for round-the-clock service for a year would cost approximately $500,000 ($$$$).

2. **Nursing registries**: Nursing registries are managed lists of nurses. In general, registries are not as selective as agencies. There usually are cost savings by using registry nurses as compared to agency nurses ($$$+).

3. **Direct hiring**: While there can be considerable cost savings, hiring a nurse directly can be difficult if you want 24-7 coverage. It can be done, but you will need to virtually form your own company with four to five nurses, given that there are 168 hours in a week and that the nurses will need time off. In addition to ensuring patient care, there will be employment issues, such as recruitment, license verification, background checks, drug testing, workers'-compensation coverage, and payroll, that you will also need to take care of. If you are going to directly hire nurses, referrals from people you know are valuable ($$$–$$$$).

Health-insurance coverage for home nursing varies considerably. Many policies do not provide any coverage. Medicare provides only very limited home nursing. One place you might not think to look is your long-term care policy. Depending on the individual long-term care policy, you may have coverage for all or part of the cost of a home caregiver working through a state-licensed registry or agency. Medicaid is an option for those patients who can't afford home care otherwise, but it can be a long process to qualify for benefits, sometimes taking a year or two. Medicaid provides some coverage for home health aides in most states.

If your family is going to care for you, they will need to know several important concepts. While I cannot provide comprehensive instructions here, important skills include the following:

1. Helping you avoid aspiration into your lungs when vomiting

2. Accurately taking your temperature

3. Moving you in bed from side to side to avoid pressure ulcers

4. Helping you avoid dehydration even if you are nauseated

5. Knowing when to use as-needed medications

6. Knowing the signs and symptoms that indicate a need to call 911 and then your doctor. They include the following:
   a. Difficulty awakening
   b. Acute confusion as compared to hours earlier
   c. Fever over a number set by the doctor
   d. Vomiting blood
   e. Shortness of breath
   f. Chest pain

Action Step Fourteen: Monitor For Depression And Anxiety, And Consider Mental Health Care

Make a point of living as optimally as possible while receiving treatment. By this I mean find a healthy balance between introspection and privacy and socializing and engagement. Avoiding or minimizing depression and anxiety is key to living fully.

Pancreatic cancer is not just a disease of the pancreas. It is also one of the most distressing stimuli to your brain and psyche imaginable. It is perfectly normal for a patient diagnosed with the disease to be distraught and even terrified. Fortunately, steps can be taken to manage anxiety and keep pancreatic cancer from causing a major depression or worsening an existing depression.[40]

We rarely think of the brain as an organ like the kidneys or liver because it is the essence of who we are: the psyche. Perhaps it would help to envision the brain as two separate things. One is the psyche. The other is the organ.

The organ can be affected by stimuli such as drugs, alcohol, and the adrenaline we produce from fear. Except to a minor degree, you cannot

---

40. Dr. Nicholas Aradi, facsimile communication to author, September 19, 2016

willfully overrule these effects. If you drink enough alcohol, you will become intoxicated. You cannot stay awake when given general anesthesia.

An analogy is a man or woman riding a horse. Think of the psyche as the person and the organ as the horse. The person is smarter, but the horse is stronger. When the person controls the horse, great things happen. A horse bucking is in a way like clinical depression. Your brain (organ) is not functioning properly. Like a rider who cannot tame a wild horse, your psyche (you) will tend to incorrectly and unmercifully blame yourself for anxiety and depression you cannot overcome without help.

Your primary care physician or oncologist should assess you for clinical depression and anxiety soon after a pancreatic cancer diagnosis. If you have had depression, anxiety or both in the past, your risk of recurrence because of pancreatic cancer is high. In this case, you should see a mental health professional right away and perhaps start medication and/or get cognitive treatment and counseling.

Major depression is a medical disease separate from pancreatic cancer. While cancer can trigger depression, it is a myth that everyone with pancreatic cancer must become depressed in the medical sense. Nonetheless, it is common. When clinical depression occurs in patients with pancreatic cancer, it can worsen the flu-like symptoms, appetite suppression, sleep disturbance, and the sadness that patients are already experiencing.

While physicians cannot currently cure metastatic pancreatic cancer, they can be successful in preventing or treating depression. Mental health services can be quite helpful in partially relieving one of most distressing side effects associated with the cancer treatment. The most successful treatment for depression is a combination of medications prescribed by a psychiatrist and counseling with a psychologist. Medications can include stimulants, antidepressants, and antianxiety drugs.

One type of counseling used by psychologists is cognitive behavioral therapy (CBT), which has the advantage of generally requiring fewer sessions than other psychological treatments. CBT focuses on encouraging awareness of your daily thoughts, especially *automatic thoughts* that may keep recurring in your mind. *Self-defeating* thoughts, such as *catastrophizing,* are one example. While having pancreatic cancer is a catastrophe in many senses, each symptom does not have to be thought of that way. While undergoing CBT, you will be taught how to consciously replace distressing thoughts with more positive thoughts and beliefs.[41]

Emotional support is very important. The people in your life will help you avoid depression and maximize your quality of life. There is a tendency for pancreatic cancer patients to isolate themselves. Sometimes, this is for a good reason, as there will be times when you will not feel well. However, there is a tendency to isolate yourself too much. This can be because you do not want to burden others or because you feel self-conscious because your looks have changed.

It is vital to most people to discuss their thoughts, fears, and wishes for the future. You will probably know intuitively whom to discuss these topics with. In addition to these conversations, I recommend that you consider seeing a psychologist even if you are not depressed. Psychologists are trained to give you not only empathy but also helpful feedback as you navigate through this difficult time.

Other ways to prevent depression are to make sure you are mentally stimulated, exercise regularly, and get adequate sleep—all of which are discussed in the next section. These are much easier said than done when dealing with the physical symptoms of pancreatic cancer and its treatment.

---

41. Ibid.

Action Step Fifteen: Living With Pancreatic Cancer

Nutrition

Correcting deficiencies with supplements generally improves health. Pancreatic enzymes that help digest food are often lacking in pancreatic cancer patients. Fortunately, they can be replaced with over-the-counter and prescription supplements. I recommend the prescription pancreatic enzymes because they have better quality control and because prescription supplements are taken at the direction of your doctor. Pancreatic cancer Action Network (PanCAN—an American nonprofit organization that funds research and provides patient support and advocacy) offers a very good and in-depth discussion of pancreatic enzymes.[42]

There is a debate about whether you should eat sugar, especially *free sugar*, while you have pancreatic cancer. Large amounts of free sugars are found in fruit juices, table sugar, honey, maple syrup, and foods made from them, such as many desserts. The sugar we eat raises the level of glucose (a type of sugar in your bloodstream) that feeds all cells. The

42. "Pancreatic Enzymes," Pancreatic Action Network, Last Modified 2017, https://www.pancan.org/facing-pancreatic cancer/diet-and-nutrition/pancreatic-enzymes/, accessed May 30, 2017.

hungriest of cells are cancer cells because they are rapidly growing. While compulsive avoidance of all sugar alone will not cure or arrest your cancer, decreasing your sugar intake is likely to be beneficial in avoiding diabetes and possibly slowing cancer cell growth.

During your disease, and especially because of chemotherapy, there will likely be times when eating and drinking enough is a struggle. Fever and profuse sweating also lead to dehydration, which can occur in only a few hours. Severe dehydration disrupts the normal chemical balance of the body. While the body tolerates mild dehydration, moderate to severe dehydration can be a serious medical problem. The Mayo Clinic shares the following information about dehydration:

Dehydration can lead to serious complications, including:

- **Heat injury.** If you do not drink enough fluids when you're exercising vigorously and perspiring heavily, you may end up with a heat injury, ranging in severity from mild heat cramps to heat exhaustion or potentially life-threatening heatstroke.

- **Urinary and kidney problems.** Prolonged or repeated bouts of dehydration can cause urinary tract infections, kidney stones, and even kidney failure.

- **Seizures.** Electrolytes—such as potassium and sodium—help carry electrical signals from cell to cell. If your electrolytes are out of balance, the normal electrical messages can become mixed up, which can lead to involuntary muscle contractions and sometimes to a loss of consciousness.

- **Low blood volume shock (hypovolemic shock).** This is one of the most serious, and sometimes life-threatening, complications of dehydration. It occurs when low blood volume causes a drop in blood pressure and a drop in the amount of oxygen in your body.[43]

To help you avoid dehydration, you can supplement your fluids with gelatin, milkshakes, and sports drinks (ones without excess caffeine) in addition to water. Should you become dehydrated to the point of dizziness when you stand up, you should call your doctor. If dehydration becomes severe, IV fluids given at home or at a medical facility will usually correct the problem but will not prevent reoccurrence.

Supplements

I am generally against the use of vitamins and other supplements if you do not have a proven deficiency. Even an unneeded multivitamin can, in some circumstances, be harmful,[44] so discuss any supplements—even just vitamins—with your oncologist. As previously discussed, the body is tremendously complex. Do not make it your own personal chemistry experiment!

Supplementation with antioxidants such vitamins A, C, and E, selenium, and zinc is particularly important to discuss with your oncologist. The scientific literature is not clear about whether these vitamins are helpful or harmful when you have pancreatic cancer. Likely, it depends on dose and the specific characteristics of your cancer.

A case in point is the multiple recommendations for megadoses of vitamin C to treat pancreatic cancer and minimize chemotherapy side effects. The recommended doses are fifty to one hundred times that of a

43. Mayo Clinic Staff, "Dehydration," Last Modified October 29, 2016, http://www.mayoclinic.org/diseases-conditions/dehydration/symptoms-causes/dxc-20261072, accessed May 30, 2017, used with the permission of Mayo Foundation for Medical Education and Research, all rights reserved.

44. Stephanie Stickel, "Why Multivitamins Might Do More Harm Than Good," Last Modified September 16, 2014, https://greatist.com/grow/why-you-dont-need-a-multivitamin, accessed July 4, 2017.

typical vitamin C tablet. The doses are so high that they can only be given by IV. This treatment has not been approved by the Food and Drug Administration. No claims that high-dose vitamin C treats or cures cancer can legally be made. Many experts are concerned that in minimizing side effects it may inactivate chemotherapy. Nonetheless, vitamin C holds some unproven promise. An in-depth discussion is made by Dr. Lichtenfeld of the American Cancer Society.[45] Dr. Heaney of Memorial Sloan Kettering published biochemical data suggesting against receiving high-dose vitamin C while receiving chemotherapy.[46] If you are interested in vitamin C therapy, definitely discuss it with your oncologist before starting.

Additional supplements to discuss with your oncologist include the following:

1. **Iron supplements**: Iron deficiency in patients with gastrointestinal cancers (pancreatic cancer is in this group) is caused by a combination of three factors, nutritional deficiencies, malabsorption, and blood loss.[47] You should be tested for iron deficiency. If you are deficient, you should take iron supplements as directed by your doctor. The goal of iron supplementation is to improve your quality of life by reducing your fatigue. Fatigue in pancreatic cancer patients is caused by many factors, so iron supplements will likely reduce but not eliminate fatigue.

---

45. Lenard J. Lichtenfeld, "Vitamin C: Have We Learned from the Past?," *Dr. Len's Blog*, Last Modified September 14, 2005, http://blogs.cancer.org/drlen/2005/09/14/vitamin-c-have-we-learned-from-the-past/, accessed May 30, 2017.

46. Mark Heany et al., "Vitamin C Antagonizes the Cytotoxic Effects of Antineoplastic Drugs," *Cancer Research* 68, no. 19 (October 2008): 8031–38, http://cancerres.aacrjournals.org/content/68/19/8031.long, accessed May 30, 2017.

47. Kristof Verraes and Hans Prenen, "Iron Deficiency in Gastrointestinal Oncology," *Annals of Gastroenterology* 28, no. 1 (2015): 19–24. https://www.ncbi.nlm.nih.gov/pmc/articles/PMC4289999/.

2. **Paricalcitol**: A special type of vitamin D that generally causes few, if any, side effects. It interferes with the ability of pancreatic cancer cells to form a fibrous layer that protects them from the immune system.[48, 49] Please note that over-the-counter vitamin D supplements do not have this effect and cannot be substituted for paricalcitol.

3. **Resveratrol**: Most of the literature shows that this supplement has a modest anti-tumor effect in pancreatic cancer. There is at least one study that raises concerns about resveratrol interfering with how chemotherapy kills cells. Another concern is that it mildly thins the blood, making bleeding slightly more likely and more difficult to control if it does occur. Even though resveratrol is a supplement that can be purchased without a prescription, it should be taken only at the direction of your oncologist. The best formulation of resveratrol is, in my opinion, transresveratrol.

4. **Multivitamins**: Again, the cardinal rule is to make sure that your oncologist recommends, or at least agrees with, your taking a multivitamin and mineral supplement. According to the American Cancer Society,[50] one should choose a multivitamin that does not exceed 100 percent of the Food and Drug Administration's recommended daily intake for each of its vitamins and minerals.

---

48. Salk Institute for Biological Studies, "Modified Vitamin D Shows Promise as Treatment for Pancreatic cancer," Last Modified September 25, 2014, http://www.salk.edu/news-release/modified-vitamin-d-shows-promise-as-treatment-for-pancreatic cancer/, accessed May 30, 2017.

49. Kerry Kaplan, *cure*, "A Promising New Treatment Offers Hope in the Fight against Pancreatic cancer," Last Modified March 10, 2016, http://www.curetoday.com/share-your-story/a-promising-new-treatment-offers-hope-in-the-fight-against-pancreatic cancer?p=2, accessed May 30, 2017.

50. "Benefitis of Good Nutrtion During Cancer Treatment," American Cancer Society, Last Modified July 15, 2015, https://www.cancer.org/treatment/survivorship-during-and-after-treatment/staying-active/nutrition/nutrition-during-treatment/benefits.html, accessed May 30, 2017.

Sleep

Insomnia and chronic fatigue frequently occur in pancreatic cancer patients. A combination of cancer symptoms, stress, and treatment side effects is the cause. Since you are probably taking several drugs, it is best to combat insomnia without the use of additional drugs, if possible. Cognitive behavioral therapy techniques are a good place to start. If this approach is not effective, ask your doctor about sleeping medicine. You will need more sleep than usual because both your cancer and its treatment drain you of energy.

Exercise

An article citing several studies of patients with breast and colon cancer found that walking "has a huge impact on survival"[51] for these patients. While not a cure in and of itself, keeping your immune system strong through mild to moderate exercise can be a meaningful part of your fight against pancreatic cancer. When possible, mild to moderate daily exercises such as walking or yoga will help with both mental and physical health.

Except when you are maximally ill, you should do a little walking every day. Walking to the kitchen or the bathroom does not count. If you are weak, just walk around the house. If you are unsteady, have someone assist you, because a fall could be a disaster. A timed walk of only three or five minutes once or twice a day may be ideal. If you are feeling normal, walk for thirty to forty-five minutes daily and add some light weights or exercise equipment every other day.

The body responds best to exercise that is continuous—over a few to many minutes—and that is frequent. For instance, six days a week is a good goal. Even though some exercise is good, more is not better. Do not maximally exert yourself, as that can weaken the immune system.

---

51. Sophie Borland, "Daily 30-Minute Walk May Slash Cancer Deaths by Half: Studies Find Regular Exercise Has a Huge Impact on Survival by Slowing Tumour Growth," *Daily Mail*, Last Modified 2017, http://www.dailymail.co.uk/news/article-4575268/Daily-30-minute-walk-slash-cancer-deaths-half.html, accessed June 6, 2017.

Summary

"Do the best you can at the time you are doing it" are the words of my grandmother, Evelina Carlson, who helped inspire this book. The goal of this book is to help you receive the best possible care currently available. It will probably not be possible for you to personally affect the progress of medical research. Rather, availing of everything that is currently known is the goal.

I advocate not simply for a multidisciplinary approach but also for these opinions to be as independent as possible. For instance, if you get the opinions of two professors of medicine or oncology, they should be at different academic medical centers. If you were to skydive, you would double-check all aspects of your parachute and your plan before you jumped. You need to proceed similarly in treating your pancreatic cancer.

Your team should, at the very least, consist of specialists in oncology, specialists in palliative medicine, and a genetic expert. Ideally, these professionals will have free and complete information exchange, but it is not a perfect world. It has been my experience that much like with the FBI, NSA, and CIA before 9/11, information exchange between medical specialists is incomplete, at best, and needs to be actively encouraged.

Your most powerful asset in this process will be your care team and your access to information. In the published scientific literature, there are glimmers of hope. Not all pancreatic cancer studies are being done in the United States. If there is an international breakthrough, it would be almost immediately known to American doctors. While I do not recommend running to the international airport on diagnosis, for some in the $$$ and $$$$ categories, medical tourism for experimental treatment may be an option.

While everyone would love a cure for pancreatic cancer, the goal in the short-run is to make pancreatic cancer non-lethal with minimal side effects. The more you can have your treatment targeted to the specifics of your cancer, the better off you are likely to be. Those with a defective DNA-mismatch-repair enzyme are, in a way, lucky. This 15 percent of patients have more and possibly better treatment options. Truly controlling cancer is probably an ongoing process of making informed and timely changes in therapy, such as those *guided by testing of an organoid*.

The fibrous stroma caused by pancreatic cancer is more important than currently appreciated. Tests to measure the amount fibrosis in each patient need to be adapted to the clinical setting from research laboratories. While this aspect of pancreatic cancer needs more study, oncologists could consider prescribing Halozyme and Paricalcitol based on the degree of fibrosis in each patient's cancer.

The hope is for targeted therapy, including personalized medicine. This tends to have fewer and less severe side effects and is becoming increasingly available. Targeted therapy is based largely on the fact that different cancer cells have different protein surfaces. It is a customized approach based on cell markers. Think of these markers as "doors" on cell surfaces. "Opening" them destroys cancer cells.

The ultimate breakthrough will probably come through genetics or immunotherapy. Genetics aided by "big data" computer analysis will probably give us an effective screening test first. Unlocking the related mysteries of genetics and the immune system is our best hope for the elusive cure(s).

There is no recipe for how to fight pancreatic cancer. I hope I have given advice general enough to accommodate the differences in patients and their needs. Meanwhile, I tried to be specific enough to give you meaningful information. On behalf of the many people who have helped me with this book, I wish you good luck and God's blessings as you fight and hopefully win your battle with pancreatic cancer.

Appendix A: Yellow Flags And Red Flags

Red Flags—Change Physicians

1. If any of your physicians are not licensed in the state where you see him or her
2. If you feel that you cannot clearly communicate with your physician despite using a medical translator
3. If your oncologist advises against getting genetic studies because "we won't know what to do with the results."
4. If your oncologist is not willing to fully participate in a team approach with fellow physicians and other professionals

Yellow Flags—Consider Changing Physicians

1. If your oncologist is guarded or defensive about discussing alternative treatments
2. If your state board of medicine has taken disciplinary action against your physician
3. If your oncologist is not board certified in hematology and oncology

4. If your oncologist's board certification in hematology and oncology has expired
5. If your oncologist does not allow generous time for questions and answers
6. If there is a language barrier between you and your oncologist

Appendix B: Resources For Further Information

Suggested Web Searches

- Pathology second opinion
- Pancreatic cancer radiology second opinion
- Best hospitals for cancer
- Remote second opinion cancer
- Pancreatic cancer organoid clinical research
- (Your state) physician license lookup

Videos

- https://www.youtube.com/watch?v=YmsR_Vmom8o (Nutrition—time range 3:43 to 4:24)
- http://www.hopkinsmedicine.org/kimmel_cancer_center/centers/pancreatic_cancer/pancreatic_cancer_videos.html (Example of an academic center offering second opinions)
- https://www.youtube.com/watch?v=DH9m-4bRYOc (About organoids, beginning at the two-minute mark for a couple of minutes—beyond then it becomes confusingly detailed)

Web Addresses

- http://www.newsweek.com/why-top-cancer-center-could-save-your-life-81425 (The first website to read—a 2009 *Newsweek* article that is still accurate and highly relevant)
- http://seer.cancer.gov/statfacts/html/pancreas.html (US government statistics about pancreatic cancer)
- http://www.aafp.org/afp/2014/1001/p476.html (Medical journal article about the use of interpreters)
- http://www.modernhealthcare.com/article/20140830/MAGAZINE/308309945 (Medical journal article about hospitals not routinely following the rule about providing qualified medical interpreters and how you might have to be assertive if you need one)
- http://pathology.jhu.edu/pc/basicheredity.php?area=ba (Johns Hopkins web page was written for the public about heredity and pancreatic cancer)
- http://jjco.oxfordjournals.org/content/32/10/391.full (Medical journal article about early symptoms of pancreatic cancer—have your family members read for themselves)

Charitable Foundations

- https://www.codepurplenow.org/
- http://lustgarten.org/homepage
- http://www.letswinpc.org/
- https://www.pancan.org/facing-pancreatic cancer/treatment/specialists/finding-a-specialist-or-cancer-center/
- http://www.seenamagowitzfoundation.org/
- http://www.standup2cancer.org/dream_teams/view/the_su2c_the_lustgarten_foundation_pancreatic_cancer_convergence_dream_team

- http://pancreatic.org/
- https://www.pancreasfoundation.org/

Website and video hyperlinks are available at Campazzi.com and are kept updated.

Appendix C: Websites To Verify Medical Licenses

Alabama http://www.albme.org/licsearchinput.html

Alaska https://www.commerce.alaska.gov/web/cbpl/ProfessionalLicensing/StateMedicalBoard/Professional-LicenseSearch.aspx

Arizona https://www.azmd.gov/glsuiteweb/clients/azbom/public/WebVerificationSearch.aspx

Arkansas https://www.armedicalboard.org/public/verify/

California http://www.mbc.ca.gov/Breeze/License_Verification.aspx

Colorado https://www.colorado.gov/dora/licensing/Lookup/LicenseLookup.aspx

Connecticut https://www.elicense.ct.gov/Lookup/LicenseLookup.aspx

Delaware https://dpronline.delaware.gov/mylicense%20weblookup/Search.aspx

Florida https://appsmqa.doh.state.fl.us/MQASearchServices/HealthCareProviders

Georgia https://services.georgia.gov/dch/mebs/jsp/index.jsp

Hawaii https://pvl.ehawaii.gov/pvlsearch/

Idaho	https://isecure.bom.idaho.gov/BOMPublic/LPRBrowser.aspx
Illinois	https://ilesonline.idfpr.illinois.gov/DPR/Lookup/LicenseLookup.aspx
Indiana	https://mylicense.in.gov/everification/Search.aspx
Iowa	https://eservices.iowa.gov/PublicPortal/Iowa/IBM/licenseQuery/LicenseQuery.jsp?Profession=Physician
Kansas	https://www.accesskansas.org/ssrv-ksbhada/search.html
Kentucky	http://web1.ky.gov/GenSearch/LicenseSearch.aspx?AGY=5
Louisiana	https://services.lsbme.org/verifications/ (Click the "I am not a robot" box and follow directions)
Maine	https://www.pfr.maine.gov/ALMSOnline/ALMSQuery/(X(1)S(w0nc4krg1symkkqsw5qpqvnp))/SearchIndividual.aspx?Board=376&AspxAutoDetectCookieSupport=1
Maryland	https://www.mbp.state.md.us/bpqapp/
Massachusetts	http://profiles.ehs.state.ma.us/Profiles/Pages/FindAPhysician.aspx
Michigan	https://w2.lara.state.mi.us/VAL/License/Search
Minnesota	https://bmp.hlb.state.mn.us/DesktopModules/ServiceForm.aspx?svid=30&mid=176
Mississippi	https://www.ms.gov/medical_licensure/renewal/verificationSearch.jsp
Missouri	https://renew.pr.mo.gov/licensee-search.asp
Montana	https://ebiz.mt.gov/pol/
Nebraska	https://www.nebraska.gov/LISSearch/search.cgi
Nevada	https://nsbme.mylicense.com/Verification/Search.aspx
New Hampshire	http://business.nh.gov/medicineboard/Disclaimer.aspx
New Jersey	https://newjersey.mylicense.com/verification_4_6/Search.aspx
New Mexico	http://docfinder.docboard.org/nm/

New York	http://www.op.nysed.gov/opsearches.htm
North Carolina	https://wwwapps.ncmedboard.org/Clients/NCBOM/Public/LicenseeInformationSearch.aspx
North Dakota	https://www.ndbom.org/public/find_verify/verify.asp
Ohio	https://license.ohio.gov/lookup/default.asp?division=78
Oklahoma	http://www.okmedicalboard.org/search
Oregon	https://techmedweb.omb.state.or.us/Clients/ORMB/Public/VerificationRequest.aspx
Pennsylvania	https://www.pals.pa.gov/#/page/search
Rhode Island	http://209.222.157.144/RIDOH_Verification/Search.aspx?facility=N&SubmitComplaint=Y
South Carolina	https://verify.llronline.com/LicLookup/Med/Med.aspx?div=16.&AspxAutoDetectCookieSupport=1
South Dakota	https://login.sdbmoe.gov/public/services/verificationsearch
Tennessee	https://apps.health.tn.gov/licensure/
Texas	https://public.tmb.state.tx.us/HCP_Search/searchinput.aspx
Utah	https://secure.utah.gov/llv/search/index.html
Vermont	https://apps.health.vermont.gov/cavu//Lookup/LicenseLookup.aspx
Virginia	https://dhp.virginiainteractive.org/Lookup/Index
Washington	https://fortress.wa.gov/doh/providercredentialsearch/
West Virginia	https://wvbom.wv.gov/public/search/
Wisconsin	https://app.wi.gov/licensesearch
Wyoming	https://wybomprod.glsuite.us/GLSuiteWeb/Clients/WYBOM/Public/Licenseesearch.aspx?SearchType=Physician

Appendix D: Definitions And Abbreviations

Amino acids: Like cement blocks are to buildings, amino acids are the building blocks of proteins. DNA instructs the sequence of the twenty types of amino acids. In turn, the sequence of the amino acids determines the function of the protein. This is like cement blocks being laid in a pattern ideal for a home which determines that this building will be used to live in.

CT (computerized tomography): Images from multiple x-rays taken at many angles. A computer interprets these x-rays together, giving three-dimensional views.

DNA (deoxyribonucleic acid): Chemical molecules that are the building blocks of genes and the instructions for every cell. Damage to DNA is the root cause of pancreatic cancer. It is a very complicated system. Fully understanding and manipulating DNA would advance treatment and early detection of pancreatic cancer.

Enzymes: These are proteins that act like robots on an assembly line. They each do one job and do it over and over again. Cell receptor proteins are like doorbells. They notify the cell when a hormone (messenger of the body) arrives. There are literally millions of examples of jobs enzymes do.

Understanding dysfunctional enzymes unique to your pancreatic cancer offers hope for better treatment.

Endoscopic ultrasound: An imaging technique using sound waves to produce images of your pancreas. Since your pancreas is near the center of your body, the probe that produces the sound wave and the microphone that records its echoes are placed near the pancreas using a tube through your mouth, down your esophagus, and into your stomach. You are given mild anesthesia for this procedure.

IV (intravenous line): This is a tiny rubber tube that drips medicine and rehydration fluid (a sterile special type of saltwater) directly into one of your veins. There are two types:

1. *Peripheral:* Inserted into a small vein (usually in the arm). It is used on a temporary basis (a few hours to a couple of days) for rehydration, antibiotics, and other medication. A peripheral IV is inserted using a needle. The needle is pulled out immediately, but the tube remains in the vein. The tube can be slightly uncomfortable when you move, giving the false sensation that the needle might remain.
2. *Central:* Often called a *port*. This is a slightly bigger tube inserted during a minor surgical procedure into a large vein—often the one under your collarbone, subclavian. It connects to about a half-inch-diameter septum that resembles the top of a drum or a bull's-eye. The septum remains entirely under your skin for months without, much if any, discomfort. This is where an IV tube can easily be inserted to deliver chemotherapy. Chemotherapy must be given into a large vein because it is so powerful that it would burn a peripheral vein, causing numerous problems.

Metastatic: Cancer that has spread by way of the bloodstream or lymphatic channels to distant parts of the body. Note that metastatic cancer still has the properties of the original cancer regardless of location. For instance, pancreatic cancer that has metastasized to the liver is still pancreatic cancer, not liver cancer.

MRCP (magnetic resonance cholangiopancreatography): An MRI with IV dye used to make detailed images of the pancreas, pancreatic duct, liver, gallbladder, and bile duct.

MRI or MR (magnetic resonance imaging): An imaging technique that uses a strong magnetic field but no radiation to produce computer-generated, three-dimensional images of the body.

Palliative care:

Palliative care (pronounced PAL-lee-uh-tiv) is specialized medical care for people with serious illness. This type of care is focused on providing relief from the symptoms and stress of a serious illness. The goal is to improve the quality of life for both the patient and the family.

Palliative care is provided by a specially trained team of doctors, nurses, and other specialists who work together with a patient's other doctors to provide an extra layer of support. It is appropriate at any age and at any stage in a serious illness, and it can be provided along with curative treatment.[52]

RNA (ribonucleic acid): A chemical the body uses in the process of taking the information stored in DNA to make proteins. Not all genes in a given cell are being used at any one time. The presence of RNA specific to a gene means that gene is active. Think of the "R" in RNA as a "receipt" for the use

---

52. GetPalliativeCare.org, https://getpalliativecare.org/whatis/, accessed May 30, 2017.

of a gene. Testing for RNA is much more expensive than testing for DNA, but it offers hope for the diagnosis and treatment of pancreatic cancer.

PERT (pancreatic enzyme replacement therapy): Oral supplements to help you digest food when your pancreas is not functioning properly.

Protein: Think of them as the buildings of the body. Just as there are many different types of buildings (homes, factories, stores, etc.), there are proteins that serve a vast variety of functions in the body (structure, muscle, enzymes, and cell markers). Proteins are made from unique combinations of about twenty amino acids, like buildings are made from cement blocks.

Targeted therapy: This is a general concept describing treatments based on a process of studying an aspect or aspects unique to your cancer and devising treatment(s) based on the results.

Afterword

Dr. **Earl Campazzi's request**: If my book helped you, please post a review on Amazon. If you read a free copy, please buy one, as only reviews from verified purchasers seem to count. Perhaps you can *pay it forward* by giving the extra copy to your oncologist for the next patient. This would significantly help me write a second book entitled *Just Diagnosed with Localized Pancreatic Cancer: Needed Steps Before Surgery*.

Dr. Allyson Ocean's request: Please report successful treatments to Let's Win PC (www.letswinpc.org).

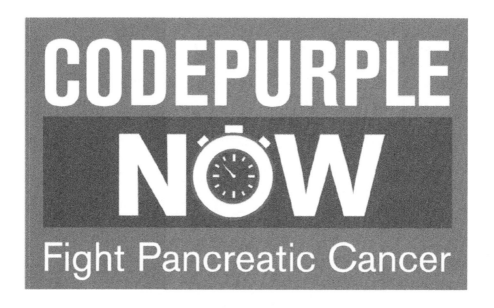

The Suzanne Wright Foundation proudly supports
Dr. Earl Campazzi and is grateful for his leadership, compassion, and com-
mitment to change the trajectory of this disease.

About The Author

Dr. Earl J. Campazzi, Jr. is board certified in four medical specialties (preventive medicine, occupational medicine, hospice/palliative medicine, and medical informatics). He has trained and practiced at some of the finest medical institutions in the country. Dr. Campazzi was on staff at the Mayo Clinic in Rochester, Minnesota, for several years. There he provided medical care to the Mayo Clinic's physicians and employees, and he was a clinical instructor at the Mayo Clinic School of Medicine. Dr. Campazzi completed his medical training at Johns Hopkins and was chosen from among a class of fourteen to be the chief resident of his program.

In addition to his medical doctorate, earned from the University of Pittsburgh School of Medicine, Dr. Campazzi has earned several postgraduate degrees. These include a master of public health degree with an emphasis in healthcare policy and management and a master of health sciences degree with an emphasis in immunology and infectious diseases, both from Johns Hopkins University Bloomberg School of Public Health. Dr. Campazzi also earned his master of business administration degree with a health-services management concentration from Duke University Fuqua School of Business. He completed his bachelor of arts degree at Johns Hopkins University.

Earl lives with his wife, Julie, in West Palm Beach, Florida. Julie is the author of a mesmerizing time-travel adventure to mythical Greece for middle-grade children. They have two dogs: Shadow (Standard Poodle) and Buster (Chinese Crested Powderpuff). They love to go on an annual cruise and to vacation in Hawaii.

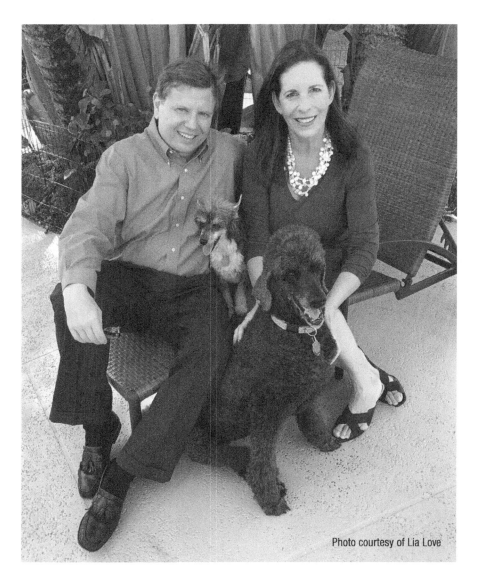

Photo courtesy of Lia Love

We wish you the best!

Made in United States
North Haven, CT
03 January 2024

46980295R00075